C0-AKB-821

# MEDICAL EVALUATION OF THE SURGICAL PATIENT

Edited by

## ALAN G. ADLER, M.D.
Clinical Assistant Professor of Medicine

with the assistance of

## GENO J. MERLI, M.D.
Clinical Assistant Professor of Medicine

## GUY E. McELWAIN, M.D.
Clinical Assistant Professor of Medicine

## JOHN H. MARTIN, M.D.
Professor of Medicine

Thomas Jefferson University, Philadelphia, Pennsylvania

## 1985

## W. B. SAUNDERS COMPANY
Philadelphia   London   Toronto   Mexico City
Rio de Janeiro   Sydney   Tokyo

Blue Books Series is a trademark of the W. B. Saunders Company.

W. B. Saunders Company:    West Washington Square
                            Philadelphia, PA   19105

                            1 St. Anne's Road
                            Eastbourne, East Sussex BN21 3UN, England

                            1 Goldthorne Avenue
                            Toronto, Ontario M8Z 5T9, Canada

                            Apartado 26370—Cedro 512
                            Mexico 4, D.F., Mexico

                            Rua Coronel Cabrita, 8
                            Sao Cristovao Caixa Postal 21176
                            Rio de Janeiro, Brazil

                            9 Waltham Street
                            Artarmon, N.S.W. 2064, Australia

                            Ichibancho, Central Bldg., 22-1 Ichibancho
                            Chiyoda-Ku, Tokyo 102, Japan

**Library of Congress Cataloging in Publication Data**
Main entry under title:

Medical evaluation of the surgical patient.

    1. Sick—Medical examination.    2. Diagnosis, Surgical.
I. Adler, Alan G.    [DNLM: 1. Preoperative Care.
2. Surgery, Operative.    WO 179 M489]
RD35.M48    1985        616'.00246171        84-22240
ISBN 0-7216-1146-X

Medical Evaluation of the Surgical Patient            ISBN   0-7216-1146-X

Last digit is the print number:      9    8    7    6    5    4    3    2    1

To our wives
Pat, Charlotte, Beth, and Martina

# CONTRIBUTORS

FREDERICK M. FELLIN, M.D.

Instructor in Medicine, Jefferson Medical College of Thomas Jefferson University; Staff Physician, Thomas Jefferson University Hospital and Wills Eye Hospital, Philadelphia, Pennsylvania.

EDWARD F. McCLAY, M.D.

Instructor in Medicine, Jefferson Medical College of Thomas Jefferson University; Fellow, Department of Oncology, Thomas Jefferson University, Philadelphia, Pennsylvania.

SANDRA F. SCHNALL, M.D.

Instructor in Medicine, Jefferson Medical College of Thomas Jefferson University, Philadelphia, Pennsylvania; Post-doctoral Fellow in Hematology and Oncology, Yale-New Haven Hospital, New Haven, Connecticut.

# GLOSSARY OF ABBREVIATIONS

| | |
|---|---|
| BP | blood pressure |
| BUN | blood urea nitrogen |
| CBC | complete blood count |
| CNS | central nervous system |
| cu mm | cubic millimeter |
| dl | deciliter |
| ECG | electrocardiographic, electrocardiogram |
| EEG | electroencephalogram |
| $F_IO_2$ | fraction of inspired oxygen |
| gm | gram |
| h | hour |
| ICU | intensive care unit |
| IM | intramuscular |
| IV | intravenous |
| kg | kilogram |
| $\mu g$ | microgram |
| mEq | milliequivalent |
| mg | milligram |
| ml | milliliter |
| NPO | nihil per os (nothing by mouth) |
| $P_{A-a}O_2$ | alveolar–arterial gradient for oxygen |
| $P_aCO_2$ | carbon dioxide pressure (tension), arterial |
| $P_AO_2$ | partial pressure of oxygen in the alveolus |
| $P_aO_2$ | oxygen pressure (tension), arterial |
| PB | barometric pressure |
| $PCO_2$ | carbon dioxide pressure (tension) |

| | |
|---|---|
| $PH_2O$ | partial pressure of $H_2O$ |
| PO | per os (by mouth) |
| $Po_2$ | oxygen pressure (tension) |
| q | quaque (every) |
| q.i.d. | quater in die (four times a day) |
| R | respiratory quotient |
| RBCs | red blood cells |
| SGOT | serum glutamic oxaloacetic transaminase |
| SGPT | serum glutamic pyruvic transaminase |
| t.i.d. | ter in die (three times a day) |
| TPN | total parenteral nutrition |
| WBCs | white blood cells |

# CONTENTS

# 1

## PREOPERATIVE MEDICAL EVALUATION

This manual has been developed to provide the medical student, the general internist, the family practitioner, and the medical subspecialist with an overview of the essentials of preoperative medical evaluation of the surgical patient. Written *for* consulting physicians *by* general internists, it presents the fundamentals of such evaluation.

The need for a truly practical manual and reference source became apparent to us when hard-to-answer questions on preoperative evaluation surfaced frequently during our own busy consultation service and when we acted as attending physicians on the residents' consultation service. Obviously, many physicians feel insecure when called on to evaluate the preoperative patient because this important aspect of medicine is not formally "taught" during medical training. Too often, information concerning such evaluation is acquired haphazardly. Furthermore, much of this information is scattered throughout the medical, surgical, and anesthesia literature and is therefore difficult to find.

Despite this lack of preparation, physicians—especially younger physicians—are frequently asked to consult on preoperative patients, and their knowledge of this subject needs to be expanded. One third to one half of a practicing internist's new patients are seen in referral or consultation[1]; the preoperative consultation that the internist performs for surgical colleagues is one of the most common types.

This book is designed to help the medical student, the house officer, and the practicing physician develop the knowledge base that is required for making logical decisions and recommendations regarding the preoperative patient. The information and guidelines offered here have been culled from the medical literature and from our own experiences during several thousand consultations at Thomas Jefferson University Hospital and Wills Eye Hospital, both in Philadelphia.

The book was developed from a syllabus that was prepared for a workshop on "Preoperative Evaluation of the Surgical Patient," first presented at the 1982 national meeting of the American College of Physicians. The deluge of requests for copies of the syllabus made it evident that there was a great deal of interest and a real need for a manual based on our syllabus format. A considerably expanded version of the earlier effort is presented in this manual. We hope it will prove to be a valuable and convenient source of information to the physician who is asked to "clear the patient for surgery."

Physicians who require more detailed information are referred to the References at the end of each chapter or to the more encyclopedic textbooks.

# GENERAL CONCEPTS: PHILOSOPHY OF THE PREOPERATIVE EVALUATION

Surgeons regularly request that patients for whom elective surgery is planned, and sometimes those who are about to have emergency surgery, be evaluated preoperatively. The reasons for this request frequently are unclear to the consulting internist; indeed, they may not be clear to the referring surgeon. Many times the request may be for a "general" medical evaluation; that is, the surgeon is concerned about what may have been missed during the surgical evaluation of the patient. At other times the medical problems are clear-cut, such as heart disease, hypertension, or diabetes mellitus, and necessitate evaluation and subsequent follow-up by an internist.

Frequently, when the internist is asked to clear a surgical patient, this is tantamount to the internist being asked to guarantee that the patient will do well and experience no complications. Such a guarantee is impossible. No physician can eliminate all risks from a surgical procedure. The results of large-scale studies of operative risk indicate that even healthy patients who undergo a simple operative procedure sometimes suffer morbidity or mortality for reasons that cannot be explained, even after thorough preoperative and postmortem examinations. However, by careful preoperative evaluation and perioperative management, it is hoped that such morbidity and mortality can be kept to a minimum. By its very nature, all surgery carries *some* risk.

The three main objectives of the internist who is asked to see a patient for evaluation before surgery are (1) to identify the patient's medical problems by using physical diagnosis, the patient's history, and laboratory studies; (2) to determine important risk factors; and (3) to bring the patient to the operating room in the best possible medical condition within the time allotted.

# CONCEPT OF THE SURGICAL TEAM

The surgical team comprises the surgeons, anesthesiologists, consulting physicians, and the referring physician. Good communication is essential for optimal patient management. Responsibility for various aspects of patient care should be clearly defined (e.g., who will write perioperative insulin orders); otherwise, management may be chaotic and erratic.

It is not the province of the consulting internist to suggest that a particular patient would benefit from local anesthesia. Selection of anesthetic agents is the responsibility of the anesthesiologist. It is inappropriate for the internist to suggest that hypoxia or hypotension should be avoided during the procedure, because no anesthesiologist would knowingly allow these to occur.

# THE PREOPERATIVE MEDICAL EXAMINATION

The request to the internist should state clearly *why* the consultation is being sought. Such statements as "preoperative evaluation" and "preoperative evaluation of diabetes mellitus and postoperative management of the diabetes" are more helpful to the consulting internist than a request for "medical consultation." The internist should write the report of consultation by hand so that no time is lost in transcribing a dictated consultation.

## History

Past medical history should include statements as to the presence or absence of diabetes, hypertension, heart disease (including angina, rheumatic heart disease, arrhythmias, and myocardial infarction), pulmonary disease, gastrointestinal disease, genitourinary disease, recent trauma, recent stroke or history of stroke, psychiatric problems, joint disease, bleeding tendencies, drug allergies, and previous surgical complications.

Recent onset or change in symptoms (e.g., chest pain) is significant and must be documented.

## Present Medications

Present medication should be listed—not just the drug, but also the dosage. It is helpful if the referring physician or surgeon asks the patient to bring a list of medications or the drugs themselves for identification. Many times it is necessary for the consulting internist to send such medications to the hospital pharmacy for identification.

A history of alcohol or recreational drug ingestion is also essential.

## Physical Examination

The report of the physical examination should include statements about the patient's *blood pressure, pulse, general health, appearance,* and *weight* and about the following parts of the body:

- *Ears, nose,* and *throat:* Note particularly whether the patient can open his mouth or has a deviated septum.
- *Lungs:* Presence of rales or wheezes and evidence of pleural effusion.
- *Heart:* Evidence of murmurs, cardiomegaly, third heart sound, *and* arrhythmias.
- *Abdomen:* Evidence of organomegaly, tenderness, or masses.
- *Joints,* including the *neck:* Decreased range of motion, chronic joint disease, such as rheumatoid arthritis or gout.
- *Neurologic:* Patient's mental status, deep tendon reflexes, pathologic reflexes, cranial nerves.

*Pelvic* and *rectal* examinations should be performed when indicated.

The chart summary should specify the patient's present medical problems, the present treatment, and the proposed treatment while hospitalized. The medical record should include the opinion of the consultant as to whether the patient is in proper medical condition for the proposed surgery, or whether a delay in the surgery would be beneficial while preoperative risks are minimized.

A standard preoperative evaluation form may be helpful so that definite positive findings are described and negative findings are indicated by checking parts of the printed form. This system has the value of indicating that information has been requested and that negative information has been obtained.

## Laboratory Studies

How many laboratory studies are pertinent to an individual case? This question must be resolved by the individual surgical team. Too many tests may only add to the patient's apprehension and expense and contribute nothing to the preoperative evaluation. On the other hand, too few laboratory studies may cause the surgical team to overlook significant medical problems. The number of laboratory tests should be agreed on by the surgical team as a whole for each surgical procedure.

If, after evaluation, the patient is found to have special problems, the consulting internist should speak directly to the attending surgeon and the anesthesiologist. It is inappropriate for the internist to "cancel the case," for this is really the prerogative of the surgeon, who may believe that the patient's best interests are served by going ahead with the surgery after consulting with the internist, even though substantial risks exist.

# THE HEALTHY PATIENT

Many patients who are admitted for elective surgery really have no underlying medical problem. Decisions concerning the need for consultation or certain laboratory tests are then the responsibility of the attending surgeon and the anesthesiologist. The internist has little to add to the surgical treatment of a healthy patient. Consultation by an internist generally is unwarranted in a patient younger than age 40 who has no underlying medical problems. Minimal evaluation for such patients should include an examination of the heart and lungs by the consulting internist, tests for fasting blood sugar, and hemoglobin studies. Further consultation or laboratory studies should be ordered specifically by the surgical team.

Management of the healthy surgical patient is discussed fully in Chapter 13, "Special Considerations."

## REFERENCE

1. Moore RA, Kammerer WS, McGlynn TJ, et al: Consultations in internal medicine: A training program resource. J Med Educ 52:323, 1977.

# 2

# CARDIOVASCULAR SYSTEM

## I. PREOPERATIVE EVALUATION

### A. PURPOSE

1. To identify and correct perioperative risk factors
2. To estimate the risk of perioperative cardiovascular complication
3. To establish familiarity with patient

The degree of urgency of the planned surgery will dictate the amount of time available for evaluation and treatment of potential risk factors. In all cases the risk of surgery must be weighed against the risk of cardiovascular complications. Weighing the risk factors can be either extremely easy or very challenging. Deciding whether to operate in an otherwise healthy 20-year-old with a perforated appendix is not hard. Deciding on the most appropriate time to operate on a 72-year-old patient with moderately severe congestive heart failure (CHF), premature ventricular contractions (PVCs), and acute bowel obstruction is considerably more difficult. A rational decision can be made only by knowing what the specific factors are that contribute to surgical risk and how soon these factors can be modified—compared with the risk of delaying the operative procedure. The decision process must, of course, include and be tempered by clinical experience and judgment. An exact numerical weighing of risks frequently is not possible. Good communication and cooperation among consulting internist, anesthesiologist, and surgeon are essential to making the most reasonable decision with the information available. *Elective* surgery should be delayed as long as necessary to bring the patient to the operating room in optimal medical condition.

## B. CLINICAL ASSESSMENT

1. History. Take a thorough history in order to identify such symptoms as chest pain and shortness of breath, which may be indicative of coronary artery disease or CHF. Note especially recent changes in previously stable symptoms. Other potentially prognostic factors that deserve inquiry are age; previous myocardial infarctions (MIs); history of cardiac arrhythmias, palpitations, or syncope; general state of health; and coexisting medical problems. A complete medication history is essential.

2. Physical examination. Note the general status of the patient. Pay particular attention to the vital signs, noting blood pressure (with positional variations), respiratory rate, pulse rate and regularity, and temperature. It is also important to note jugular venous distention, carotid and peripheral pulses (with auscultation for bruits), presence of rales or pleural effusion, cardiac rhythm irregularities, gallops, murmurs, rubs, and edema. Check for signs of chronic liver disease or other chronic illness, and determine the general state of debilitation.

3. Laboratory studies

   a. Chest x-ray: To evaluate lung disease, cardiac enlargement, CHF

   b. Electrocardiography: To help identify conduction abnormalities, rhythm disturbance, ischemia or previous infarction, alterations secondary to electrolyte abnormalities or drugs

   c. CBC: To detect alterations in hemoglobin concentration and hematocrit, which may impair cardiac oxygen supply. Leukocyte abnormalities may be indicative of infection.

   d. Chemistries

      (1) Glucose: To rule out undiagnosed diabetes and determine status of control in the known diabetic. Hyperglycemia may result in dehydration and poor tissue perfusion. Hypoglycemia may result in increased symptomatic activity. Both may increase cardiac stress.

      (2) Electrolytes: To evaluate abnormalities that may contribute to cardiac arrhythmias or conduction defects

      (3) BUN, creatinine, liver enzymes: To detect underlying hepatic or renal disease, which may contribute to risk of surgery and increased drug toxicity. These conditions must be evaluated preoperatively.

e. Other studies: If routine assessment suggests abnormalities, further evaluation (e.g., exercise stress testing, echocardiography, electrophysiologic studies, cardiac catheterization) may be indicated before surgery.

## II. CARDIOVASCULAR RISK ESTIMATION

### A. MULTIVARIATE ANALYSIS OF RISK

A considerable number of perioperative cardiac complications are related to cardiac disease. Goldman and co-workers[1,2] have devised a scale to predict cardiac risk factors based on multivariate analyses in non-cardiac surgery.

1. Goldman et al. studied 1001 consecutive patients over age 40 undergoing general, orthopedic, or urologic surgery. Transurethral prostatectomies, endoscopies, and minor surgery were excluded.

2. Analyzed variables included sex, age, body build, dyspnea, orthopnea, edema, angina, MI by history, New York Heart Association symptomatic class, history of specific arrhythmias, diabetes, hypertension, hyperlipidemia, tobacco use, preoperative systolic and diastolic blood pressures, jugular venous distention, systolic and diastolic murmurs, hemodynamically significant valvular aortic stenosis, third or fourth heart sounds, rales, peripheral pulses, ECG rhythm, QRS axis, P–R interval, voltage, ST segments, T waves, P waves, Q waves, R wave progression, bundle-branch blocks, heart size, pulmonary vasculature, and aortic shadow by x-ray. Also considered were all available preoperative, laboratory data, signs of chronic liver disease, CNS status, known cancer, ability to care for one's own needs, type of operation, type of anesthesia, emergency or elective procedure, and training level of the surgeon.

3. Nine of the above factors were found to have a statistically significant independent correlation with cardiac outcome. These factors were weighed and given a point value based on their individual predictive values (Table 2–1).

4. A scale was then devised, based on total point values, that separated the patients into four categories of risk (Table 2–2). Obviously, all but essential surgery should be avoided in Group IV patients.

5. Further analyses of the cardiac risk factors demonstrate valuable clinical information. The pooled results of these studies demonstrate how the risk of cardiac death or recurrent MI decreases as the time between preoperative

TABLE 2–1. Index of Cardiac Risk Factors

| Criteria | Risk Factor | Points |
|---|---|---|
| History | Over age 70 | 5 |
| | MI in previous six months | 10 |
| Physical examination | Jugular venous distention or $S_3$ gallop | 11 |
| | Hemodynamically significant valvular aortic stenosis | 3 |
| Electrocardiography | Any rhythm other than sinus or PACs on last electrocardiogram before surgery | 7 |
| | More than five PVCs per minute documented on any presurgical ECG | 7 |
| General status | $Po_2 < 60$ mm Hg or $Pco_2 > 50$ mm Hg $K^+ < 3.0$ mEq/L or $HCO_3^- < 20$ mEq/L Creatinine $> 3.0$ mg/dl or BUN $> 50$ mg/dl Abnormal SGOT; signs of chronic liver disease Patient bedridden from non-cardiac causes | 3 |
| Type of operation | Emergency procedure | 4 |
| | Aortic, intrathoracic, or intraperitoneal surgery | 3 |
| | Possible total: | 53 |

Adapted from Goldman L, et al: Multifactorial index of cardiac risk in noncardiac surgical procedures. N Engl J Med 297:845–850, 1977.

MI and surgery increases. These risks may be as high as 31 per cent if surgery is performed within three months of an MI. The risk decreases to about 5 per cent to 6 per cent after six months, stabilizing thereafter (see Fig. 2–1).

TABLE 2–2. Cardiac Risk Scale

| Risk Level | Total Points | No or Minor Complications (%) | Life-threatening* Complications (%) | Cardiac Death (%) |
|---|---|---|---|---|
| I | 0–5 | 99 | 0.7 | 0.2 |
| II | 6–12 | 93 | 5 | 2 |
| III | 13–25 | 86 | 11 | 2 |
| IV | Over 26 | 22 | 22 | 56 |

Adapted from Goldman L, et al: Multifactorial index of cardiac risk in noncardiac surgical procedures. N Engl J Med 297:845–850, 1977.
*Myocardial infarction, ventricular tachycardia, pulmonary empyema

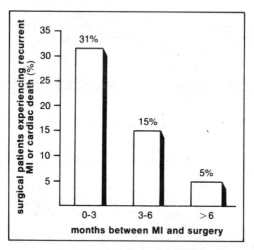

**Figure 2–1.** Relationship of new cardiac events to timing of surgery after MI. Pooled results of three recent studies show that the risk of cardiac death or recurrent myocardial infarction decreases significantly as the time increases between a preoperative MI and surgery. (From Goldman L: Guidelines for evaluating and preparing the cardiac patient for general surgery. J Cardiovasc Med 5:637–644, 1980.)

Age is not an independent risk factor until age 70, when it dramatically increases in a linear fashion (see Fig. 2–2).

As seen in Figure 2–3, intrathoracic, intra-abdominal, and aortic operations carry a higher risk in all categories of cardiac complications (death, MI, CHF, supraventricular tachycardia) compared with other major surgery.

It is important for the medical consultant to be aware that the peak onset time of MI is from the fourth to sixth day postoperatively. For this reason, extended surveillance, past the immediate postoperative period, is important (see Fig. 2–4).

## B. ADDITIONAL CARDIAC-RELATED CONSIDERATIONS (NOT INCLUDED IN THE GOLDMAN ANALYSES)

1. Angina and cardiac disease
   a. Although Goldman et al. did not demonstrate increased risk with stable angina, other studies clearly indicate an increased risk for the angina patient.

Overall mortality from combined series in the literature is about 8.7 per cent for angina patients (stability unspecified) to about 10 per cent of all heart disease patients.[4]

b. The incidence of postoperative MI is about 6 per cent in all patients with previous infarcts, compared with 0.13 per cent to 0.7 per cent of patients without known disease.[5, 6] A 50 per cent mortality can be expected in patients with a history of infarction who suffer postoperative MI.

c. Few hard data are available on unstable angina because patients rarely are subjected to non-cardiac surgery if this pattern is recognized. However, the

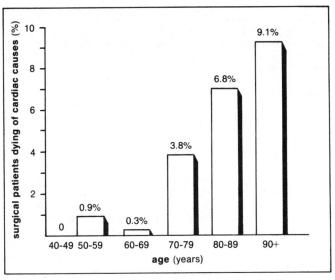

**Figure 2–2.** Relationship of patient's age to risk of perioperative cardiac death. After age 70, the risk of cardiac death associated with surgery increases in a statistically significant linear fashion. (From Goldman L: Guidelines for evaluating and preparing the cardiac patient for general surgery. J Cardiovasc Med 5:637–644, 1980.)

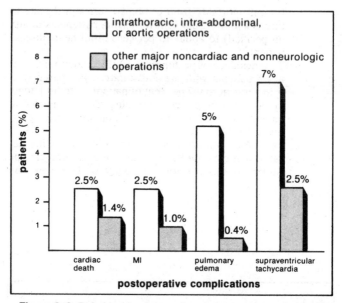

**Figure 2–3.** Relationship of type of surgery to postoperative cardiac complications. Intrathoracic, intra-abdominal, and aortic operations are associated with increased risks of both fatal and nonfatal postoperative cardiac complications. (From Goldman L: Guidelines for evaluating and preparing the cardiac patient for general surgery. J. Cardiovasc Med 5:637–644, 1980.)

mortality might be comparable to a recent MI, based on the known high mortality even without surgery.

d. Patients who have undergone coronary artery bypass surgery have less risk for subsequent non-cardiac surgery than do patients with coronary artery disease. In the largest series in the literature, by Crawford and associates,[7] the percentage of perioperative MI was 1.2 per cent, the percentage of perioperative mortality was 1.1 per cent, and serious arrhythmias developed in 2.9 per cent of 35 patients. Because 75 per cent of deaths occurred in patients undergoing the second procedure within 30 days of cardiac surgery, timing appears to be critical. However, more serious disease, necessitating surgery shortly after coronary artery bypass grafting, may have contributed to the higher mortality, rather than the risk being purely a function of timing.

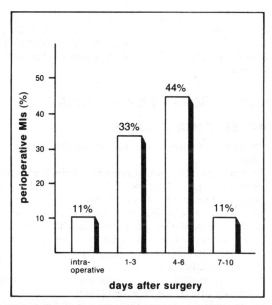

**Figure 2–4.** Onset time of perioperative myocardial infarctions. The peak risk period for perioperative myocardial infarction is from the fourth through the sixth day after surgery. (From Goldman L: Guidelines for evaluating and preparing the cardiac patient for general surgery. J Cardiovasc Med 5:637–644, 1980.)

2. Mitral valvular disease
   a. Mortality for all patients with hemodynamically significant mitral stenosis is about 5 per cent; complications of atrial fibrillation and CHF may increase mortality to as high as 20 per cent. These complications may be a marker of severer underlying disease, as well as having serious hemodynamic consequences. Complete preoperative evaluation and return to cardiac compensation are critical.

## III. RATIONALE FOR CORRECTION OF RISK FACTORS

Potentially, most risk factors can be modified, but are morbidity and mortality significantly affected? Although prospective controlled studies in this area are lacking, therapeutic logic and clinical experience support therapeutic strategies that are aimed at correcting cardiovascular factors. For example, patients with symptomatic coronary artery disease tolerate surgery far better when cardiac status is meticulously controlled. Mortality of 2 per cent or lower after coronary artery bypass has been reported at major centers.

# IV. MODIFICATION OF RISK FACTORS

## A. CONGESTIVE HEART FAILURE

1. Postpone all surgery except for life-threatening conditions.
2. Treat aggressively with diuretics and digitalis while closely monitoring jugular venous distention, weight, cardiac rate, renal function, and electrolytes.
3. Digitalis treatment and *levels* help return the patient to cardiac compensation while avoiding the hazards of excessive diuresis. Digitalis levels must be used only as a guide in conjunction with clinical assessment.
4. Prophylactic digitalis
   a. Recommended only for patients with a documented history of CHF or tachyarrhythmias.
   b. No evidence that prophylactic use of digitalis prevents CHF and arrhythmias when no preoperative clinical indications are present. Risk increases for postoperative digitalis toxicity and complicates the diagnosis and therapy of postoperative arrhythmias.
5. To achieve optimal control of fluid status, Swan-Ganz monitoring in patients with CHF who must undergo emergency surgery is essential. Patients with borderline cardiac status undergoing major elective surgery may also benefit from preoperative optimization with Swan-Ganz catheterization.

## B. RECENT MYOCARDIAL INFARCTION

1. Follow-up the patient for at least six months before any elective surgical procedure.
2. If the patient is unstable and surgery is mandatory, an intra-aortic balloon pump may be considered in order to maximize cardiac support.

## C. UNSTABLE ANGINA

1. Careful observation and postponement of nonemergent surgery is essential while maximizing medical therapy with nitrates, beta blockers, and calcium channel blockers.

2. If medical management is unsuccessful, evaluate for coronary artery bypass surgery before elective non-cardiac surgery. As noted earlier, coronary artery bypass may lower the risk of subsequent non-cardiac surgery.
3. As in the case of recent MI, if surgery cannot be postponed, intra-aortic balloon pumps may aid cardiac support.

## D. VALVULAR AORTIC STENOSIS

1. Because valvular aortic stenosis is a cardiac risk factor, it should be considered in patients with aortic valve calcifications, diminished carotid upstroke, poststenotic aortic dilatation, or left ventricular hypertrophy that is otherwise unexplained. Symptoms of angina, syncope, or CHF might be secondary to aortic stenosis as well as to many other etiologies and should be evaluated preoperatively. Murmur quality is undependable, since it might be quite diminished in tight stenosis.
2. If the patient is found to have tight aortic stenosis, priority should be given to valve replacement before elective surgery.
3. If surgery is nonelective, and if valve replacement is impossible, hemodynamic monitoring with a Swan-Ganz catheter should be considered during the perioperative period.
4. Because borderline cardiac compensation often coexists, fluid therapy must be carefully managed and monitored. Large bolus infusions should be avoided.

## E. ARRHYTHMIAS

1. Premature ventricular contractions
   a. Despite the findings of Goldman and co-workers[1,2] that preoperative ECGs showing five or more PVCs per minute were associated with increased cardiac mortality in surgery, the significance of PVCs remains controversial—particularly if the patient is asymptomatic. Ventricular ectopy must be evaluated in terms of frequency, complexity, and the patient's overall clinical status.
   b. PVCs may have their major significance as a marker of underlying heart disease, but they do not necessarily indicate a high likelihood of intraoperative or postoperative ventricular tachycardia.[8]
   c. Each clinician must use his own clinical judgment. Table 2–3 offers a reasonable approach to the evaluation and treatment of patients with PVCs.

**TABLE 2–3.    Evaluation of Patient with Premature Ventricular Contractions**

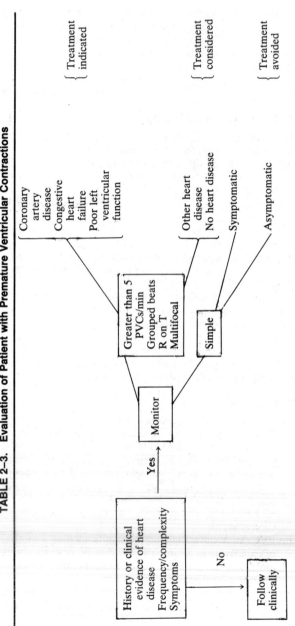

*Modified from Whiting, RB: Ventricular premature contractions. Which should be treated? Arch Intern Med *140*:1423–1426, 1980.

    d. Conventional antiarrhythmic therapy should be continued up to and through surgery for patients already under treatment, aided by appropriate drug levels (digoxin, quinidine, procainamide, and disopyramide being the most commonly available) when indicated.

2. Atrial arrhythmias (fibrillation, flutter, premature atrial contractions) and supraventricular tachycardia

    a. Evaluation of atrial arrhythmias must be directed to the underlying cause. Cardiac etiologies, including underlying valvular or congenital heart disease, cardiomyopathy, pericarditis, myocardial ischemia, CHF, sick sinus syndrome, and Wolff-Parkinson-White syndrome, must be considered as well as non-cardiac etiologies, including pulmonary embolus, infection, metabolic abnormalities (apathetic hyperthyroidism is commonly overlooked in the elderly), drug toxicity, stress, and paroxysmal idiopathic arrhythmias. These should be readily evident from a thorough history and physical examination.

    b. Treatment is aimed at maintaining hemodynamic stability and correcting the underlying disorder if possible.

       (1) Heart rate must be well controlled, since it is such an important determinant of cardiac output, particularly in atrial fibrillation. Standard digitalis or beta-blocker regimens should be used and continued throughout the perioperative period.

       (2) If the patient is hemodynamically unstable, direct-current cardioversion is indicated. For the stable patient, an attempt at chemical cardioversion is often preferred, particularly if the supraventricular dysrhythmia is of recent onset.

    c. The potential for bradyarrhythmias also needs to be considered in the patient with supraventricular arrhythmias. Sick sinus syndrome is a common etiology, particularly in the elderly patient without other obvious cause. Assessment by ambulatory or in-hospital monitoring is crucial preoperatively, since treatment with digoxin or beta blockers in combination with the negative chronotropic effects of some anesthetic agents in the patient with sick sinus syndrome may result in life-threatening bradycardia and hypotension.

    d. Anticholinergic drugs, commonly used in drug anesthesia, may precipitate an episode of tachyarrhythmias or increased heart rate in the patient with a history of tachyarrhythmia. Generally, they should be avoided whenever possible.

# V. MANAGEMENT OF OTHER IMPORTANT CARDIAC-RELATED FACTORS

## A. HYPERTENSION

1. Recent studies have demonstrated that mild to moderate hypertension is not a significant factor in determining cardiac risk.
2. Goldman and Caldera studied 676 consecutive operations in patients over age 40.[9] Their findings are as follows:
   a. Although there were greater absolute intraoperative blood pressure decreases among patients who had persistent hypertension as compared with those who had tightly controlled hypertension, the preoperative in-hospital systolic and diastolic blood pressure values of patients with hypertension histories did not independently correlate with:
      (1) intraoperative systolic pressure nadir
      (2) the use of a fluid challenge or adrenergic agent to maintain intraoperative blood pressure
      (3) the development of hypertensive events
   b. In terms of new perioperative hypertensive events, the only positive correlation was with patients who had histories of severer pre-hospital increases regardless of preoperative in-hospital control.
   c. Although Goldman and Caldera's data did not show increased risk despite larger absolute decreases in blood pressure in untreated or inadequately treated hypertensive patients, other studies have correlated large blood pressure drop with increased risk. Mauney and associates[10] reported a correlation between intraoperative blood pressure decreases of 33 per cent for longer than ten minutes and postoperative cardiac complications. Prys-Roberts et al.[11] also found ECG evidence for myocardial ischemia when mean arterial pressures decreased to 50 per cent of preoperative levels. Differences between the findings of Goldman and Caldera, and Prys-Roberts et al. may reflect not only the severer hypertension in the latter study (mean preoperative systolic pressure of 211 torr and mean preoperative diastolic pressure of 105 torr), but also the anesthesiologic ability to prevent marked intraoperative blood pressure decreases.
3. Goldman and Caldera's findings argue against the need for tight preoperative blood pressure control and suggest that:
   a. Perioperative blood pressure lability may be as much

a function of a patient's inherent vascular characteristics as of any modification of such characteristics by
antihypertensive medications.

    b. Effective intraoperative management may be more
important than preoperative hypertension control in
terms of decreasing clinically significant blood pressure
lability and cardiovascular complications in patients
with mild to moderate hypertension.

4. Current recommendations based on the results of recent
studies can be summarized as follows: Operations in
which ideal control is lacking may be performed without
increased risk if:

    a. Diastolic blood pressure is stable and not higher than
110 torr

    b. Intraoperative and recovery room blood pressures are
monitored closely and treated to prevent hypertensive
or hypotensive episodes, especially decreases to less
than 50 per cent of peoperative values or decreases of
33 per cent for longer than ten minutes

5. Antihypertensive medication

    a. Antihypertensive medication should, for the most
part, be continued up to the time of surgery, since
abrupt withdrawal of nearly all types may result in
severe rebound hypertension and beta-blocker withdrawal may result in an acute coronary event (see
later discussion).

    b. *Overaggressive* treatment with diuretics for mild to
moderate hypertension should be avoided, since (1)
mild to moderate hypertension (diastolic BP < 110)
does not increase surgical risk; (2) hypovolemia induced by diuretics may greatly exaggerate the hypotensive effects of anesthetics; (3) hypokalemia may
result.

    c. Ideally, all hypertensive patients, particularly those
with severe hypertension, should be identified and
treated adequately before hospitalization for elective
surgery. This is because at the high end of the scale
untreated or inadequately treated hypertensive patients have been shown to have larger absolute decreases in blood pressure during anesthesia than do
adequately treated patients.

## B. CARDIAC CONDUCTION DEFECTS AND PACEMAKERS

1. Consider reversible etiologies for the heart block, such
as digitalis, antiarrhythmic agents, and tricyclic antide-

pressants. Remember thât although first-degree heart block is generally benign, it may be an indicator of early digitalis toxicity. Levels should be checked.

2. No treatment is indicated for:
   a. Uncomplicated first-degree AV block
   b. Asymptomatic bifascicular block—e.g., right bundle branch block + left anterior hemiblock, right bundle branch block + right posterior hemiblock, left bundle branch block, or bifascicular block + prolonged P-R interval. In Belloci's surgical series of 98 patients with bifascicular block, there was not one documented case of complete heart block.[12]

3. A temporary or permanent pacemaker is indicated in:
   a. Mobitz II second-degree AV block, as this often progresses to complete heart block
   b. Third-degree (complete) heart block. Vandam and McLemare reported postoperative cardiac arrest in 1 of 11 patients with asymptomatic complete heart block and 5 of 11 patients with syncope and complete heart block.[13]
   c. Possibly symptomatic bifascicular block, since this may result from an intermittent higher-degree block.

4. Treatment for patients with Mobitz I second-degree AV block (Wenckebach) must be individualized, depending on etiology and symptoms.

5. Patients with programmable pacemakers may benefit from increased rate to enhance cardiac output or suppress tachyarrhythmias.

6. Electrocautery must be used with great caution, since it may temporarily suppress demand pacemaker function. Cauterization units should be kept as far from the pacemaker as possible. Patients obviously should be monitored closely, and a magnet should be available for pacemaker conversion to a fixed mode if the demand function is suppressed.

## C. BETA-BLOCKING AGENTS

1. Beta blockers are an integral part of the medical regimen for many patients with such conditions as angina, hypertension, arrhythmias, and hypertrophic cardiomyopathy.

2. Although early reports suggested a high rate of cardiac failure in patients undergoing surgery on propranolol,[14] subsequent clinical studies have not shown increased risk.[15, 16]

3. The withdrawal syndrome, consisting of worsening angina, arrhythmias, hypertension, infarction, and possibly

death, is a real concern, although not as common as generally thought.[17] Appearance of withdrawal rebound symptoms peak about four to seven days after drug discontinuation.[18]

4. Continuation of beta blockers up to the time of surgery appears safe from an anesthetic viewpoint and may help postpone the withdrawal syndrome until after oral propranolol therapy can be restarted. One recommended approach is given in Table 2–4.

5. IV propranolol infusion might be indicated in various clinical situations, such as prolonged GI tract dysfunction secondary to abdominal surgery, severe thyrotoxicosis, and acute aortic dissection. Smulyan and co-workers[19] have found that therapeutic serum propranolol levels were attained with a narrow dose range averaging 3 mg/h in patients with normal hepatic and renal function undergoing abdominal surgery. This schedule protected against sympathetic stimulation during the perioperative period and prevented the withdrawal syndrome.

## D. CALCIUM CHANNEL BLOCKERS

1. Calcium channel blockers, such as verapamil, nifedipine, and diltiazem, are relatively new drugs used in the treatment of cardiovascular disease.

2. No controlled studies have been conducted to demonstrate whether these drugs should be discontinued before anesthesia. Our experience and that of others[20] is that they may be continued safely right up to the morning of surgery.

3. Nifedipine and verapamil are potent vasodilators and must be administered cautiously in the preoperative period, especially in the presence of hypovolemia or impaired ventricular function.

4. Verapamil and diltiazem may have significant blocking effects on the AV node and must be used carefully in patients undergoing anesthesia or in those maintained on beta-adrenergic blocking drugs or digoxin.

5. Table 2–5 summarizes the pharmacologic cardiac effects of these drugs.

## E. HYPERTROPHIC CARDIOMYOPATHY

1. Patients with hypertrophic cardiomyopathy (idiopathic hypertrophic subaortic stenosis; asymmetric septal hypertrophy) are at risk for cardiac outflow obstruction and complications, including arrhythmias, heart pain, CHF, and sudden death.

**TABLE 2–4. Perioperative Propranolol Therapy***

| Indication | Preoperative Rx | Operative Rx | Postoperative Rx |
|---|---|---|---|
| Angina | Continue propranolol to morning of surgery. | IV propranolol rarely required. | Resume propranolol orally or through nasogastric tube when GI tract is functioning. Nitrates as indicated, IV propranolol for withdrawal symptoms. |
| Hypertension | Continue propranolol to morning of surgery; may be tapered 24 to 48 hours preoperatively if diastolic pressure does not exceed 110 torr. | IV nitroprusside, followed by IV methyldopa if hypertension severe. Rarely need IV propranolol. | Resume oral or nasogastric propranolol when hemodynamically stable; IV methyldopa or IM hydralazine based on severity of hypertension, if needed. |

Modified from Goldman, L: Non-cardiac surgery in patients receiving propranolol. Arch Intern Med *141*:193–196, 1981.

TABLE 2–5. Effects of Calcium Channel Blockers

| Cardiac Function | Verapamil | Nifedipine | Diltiazem |
|---|---|---|---|
| SA node automaticity | ↓ ↓ | O | ↓ |
| AV node conduction | ↓ ↓ ↓ | O/ ↓ | ↓ ↓ |
| Myocardial contractility | ↓ ↓ | ↓ | ↓ |
| Peripheral vascular resistance | ↓ ↓ | ↓ ↓ ↓ | ↓ |
| Heart rate | ↑ ↓ | ↑ | O/ ↓ |
| Cardiac output | ↓ ↑ | ↑ | O/ ↑ |

2. Important aspects of perioperative management include:
   a. Careful fluid management to prevent volume contraction and exacerbation of outflow obstruction
   b. Avoidance of inotropic agents
   c. Rapid control of arrhythmias by cardioversion, if unstable, or by propranolol, which is the drug of choice
   d. All symptomatic patients should be treated with propranolol and consideration given to perioperative hemodynamic monitoring, as should asymptomatic patients with significant obstruction or ectopy.

## F. ANTIBIOTIC PROPHYLAXIS

1. Primary and consulting physicians frequently are required to make recommendations for prophylaxis of bacterial endocarditis before surgery. They must be acquainted with the indications and treatment regimens.
2. Prophylaxis recommended for the following disorders:
   a. Valvular heart disease
   b. Congenital heart disease
   c. Prosthetic valves
   d. Previous endocarditis
   e. Mitral valve prolapse
   f. Idiopathic hypertrophic subaortic stenosis
3. Types of surgery
   a. Dental
   b. Upper respiratory tract
   c. Gastrointestinal
   d. Genitourinary tract
4. Percentage of patients developing bacteremia after specific procedures is listed in Table 2–6.
5. Current recommended prophylaxis is listed in Table 2–7.

**TABLE 2-6. Risk of Bacteremia**

| High Risk | Intermediate Risk | Low Risk |
|---|---|---|
| Prostatectomy—infected urine | Prostatectomy—sterile urine | Sigmoidoscopy 2–10% |
| Transurethral 58% | Transurethral 11% | Colonoscopy 3–6% |
| Retropubic 82% | Retropubic 13% | Eosphageal dilatation, |
| Esophageal dilatation, unsterile dilator | Barium enema 11% | sterile dilator 0% |
| 100% | Liver biopsy 3–13% | Fiberoptic bronchoscopy 0% |
| Tonsillectomy 28–38% | Rigid bronchoscopy 15% | Orotracheal intubation 0% |
| Dental extraction 18–85% | Nasotracheal intubation 16% | Parturition 0–5% |
| Periodontal surgery 21–88% | Nasotracheal suctioning, intensive-care | IUD insertion 0% |
| Burn surgery 46% | patients 16% | |
| Surgery of infected areas 54% | | |

From Flynn, N.M., and Lawrence, R.M.: Antimicrobial prophylaxis. *In* Symposium on medical evaluation of the preoperative patient. Med Clin North Am 63:1230, 1979.

**TABLE 2–7. Prophylaxis of Bacterial Endocarditis in Adults***

*Dental Procedures and Surgery of the Upper Respiratory Tract*

REGIMEN A
1. *Combined oral–parenteral penicillin*—aqueous crystalline penicillin G (1,000,000) units IM) *mixed with* procaine penicillin G (600,000 units M). Give 30 minutes to 1 hour prior to procedure and follow with penicillin V 500 mg p.o. q 6h for 8 doses.
2. *Oral penicillin*—penicillin V, 2.0 grams p.o. 30 minutes to 1 hour prior to procedure followed by 500 mg p.o. q 6h for 8 doses.
3. *For patients allergic to penicillin*—erythromycin 1.0 gram 1½–2 hours prior to procedure followed by 500 mg p.o. q 6h for 8 doses *or* vancomycin (see Regimen B).

REGIMEN B†
1. *Penicillin plus streptomycin*—aqueous crystalline penicillin G (1,000,000 units IM) *mixed with* procaine penicillin G (600,000 units IM).

*plus*

Streptomycin (1 gram IM). Give 30 minutes to 1 hour prior to procedure and follow with penicillin V 500 mg p.o. q 6h for 8 doses.
2. *For patients allergic to penicillin*—vancomycin (1 gram IV over 30 minutes to 1 hour) started 30 minutes to 1 hour prior to procedure and followed by erythromycin 500 mg p.o. q 6h for 8 doses.

*Gastrointestinal and Genitourinary Surgery and Instrumentation*

1. Aqueous crystalline penicillin G (2,000,000 units IM or IV)
   *or*
   Ampicillin (1.0 gram IM or IV)
   *plus*
   Gentamicin (1.5 mg/kg not to exceed 80 mg IM or IV)
   *or*
   Streptomycin (1.0 gram IM)
2. *For patients allergic to penicillin*—vancomycin (1.0 gram IV given over 30 minutes to 1 hour) *plus* streptomycin (1.0 gram IM). Give one dose 30 minutes prior to procedure; may repeat in 12 hours.

From Medical evaluation of the preoperative patient. Med Clin North Am *63*:1230, 1979.
   *Recommendations of the Committee on Prevention of Rheumatic Fever and Bacterial Endocarditis of the American Heart Association.
   †Regimen B is recommended for patients with prosthetic heart valves.

## G. ANTICOAGULATION THERAPY IN PATIENTS WITH PROSTHETIC HEART VALVES

1. Aortic valve
   a. Cessation of sodium warfarin for 3 to 5 days (and possibly longer) appears safe in patients with isolated aortic prosthesis.[22, 23] No cases of thromboembolism have been reported in the perioperative period with short-term interruption.
   b. Anticoagulation with sodium warfarin can be stopped 72 hours preoperatively and restarted 48 hours postoperatively.
2. Mitral valve (alone or in combination)
   a. Although rare, a small risk of thromboembolism exists in patients with mitral or combined prosthetic valves.
   b. One recommended protocol is to reverse the warfarin effect just prior to the operation and then initiate heparin therapy 12 to 24 hours after the procedure, provided that adequate hemostasis has occurred. Prior to discharge, oral anticoagulation with sodium warfarin is resumed and heparin discontinued.[23]
   c. Our procedure is to discontinued sodium warfarin 72 hours preoperatively (without specific reversal), and initiate heparin therapy 12 to 24 hours after the procedure. Sodium warfarin can then be resumed.

## *REFERENCES*

1. Goldman L, et al: Multifactorial index of cardiac risk in non-cardiac surgical procedures. N Engl J Med 297:845, 1977.
2. Goldman L, et al: Cardiac risk factors and complications in non-cardiac surgery. Medicine 57:357, 1978.
3. Goldman L: Guidelines for evaluating and preparing the cardiac patient for general surgery. J Cardiovasc Med 5:637, 1980.
4. Mollitch MD: Management of Medical Problems in Surgical Patients. Philadelphia, FA Davis, 1982, p 81.
5. Tarhan S, et al: Myocardial infarction after general anesthesia. JAMA 220:1451, 1972.
6. Knapp RB, Topkins MJ, Artusio JF: The cerebrovascular accident and coronary occlusion in anesthesia. JAMA, 182:106, 1962.
7. Crawford ES, et al: Operative risk in patients with previous coronary artery bypass. Ann Thorac Surg 26:215, 1978.
8. Whiting RB: Ventricular premature contractions. Which should be treated? Arch Intern Med 140:1423, 1980.
9. Goldman L, Caldera DL: Risk of general anesthesia and elective operations in the hypertensive patient. Anesthesiology 50:285, 1979.

10. Mauney FM, Ebert PD, Sabiston DC Jr: Post-operative myocardial infarction: A study of predisposing factors, diagnosis and mortality in a high risk group of surgical patients. Ann Surg *172*:497, 1970.

11. Prys-Roberts C, Meloche R, Foëx P: Studies of anesthesia in relation to hypertension: I. Cardiovascular responses of treated and untreated patients. Br J Anaesth *43*:112, 1971.

12. Bellocci F, Santarelli P, DiGennaro M, et al: The risk of cardiac complications in surgical patients with bifascicular block: A clinical and electrophysiologic study in 98 patients. Chest *77*:343, 1980.

13. Vandam LP, McLemare GA Jr: Circulatory arrest in patients with complete heart block during anesthesia and surgery. Am J Med *47*:518, 1957.

14. Viljoen JF, Estafanous FG, Kellner GA: Propranolol and cardiac surgery. J Thorac Cardiovasc Surg *64*:826, 1972.

15. Moran JM, Mulet J, Caralps JM, et al: Coronary revascularization in patients receiving propranolol. Circulation *50*(suppl 2): 116, 1974.

16. Kaplan JA, Dunbar RW, Bland JW Jr, et al: Propranolol and cardiac surgery: A problem for the anesthesiologist? Anesth Analg *54*:571, 1975.

17. Shand DG, Wood AJJ: Propranolol withdrawal syndrome—why? Circulation *58*:202, 1978.

18. Goldman L: Non-cardiac surgery in patients receiving propranolol. Arch Intern Med *141*:193, 1981.

19. Smilyan H, Weinberg SE, Howanitz PJ: Continuous propranolol infusion following abdominal surgery. JAMA *247*:2539, 1982.

20. Reves JG, Kissin I, Lell WA, Tosone S: Calcium channel blockers: Uses and implications for anesthesiologists. Anesthesiology *57*:504, 1982.

21. Medical Evaluation of the Preoperative Patient. Med Clin North Am *63*(5), Nov., 1979.

22. Tinker JH, Tarhan S: Discontinuing anticoagulant therapy in surgical patients with cardiac valve prostheses. JAMA *239*:738, 1978.

23. Katholi RE, Nolan SP, McGuire LB: Living with prosthetic heart valves—subsequent noncardiac operations and the risk of thromboembolism or hemorrhage. Am Heart J *92*:162, 1976.

## I. PREOPERATIVE EVALUATION

### A. PURPOSE

1. To determine the type and severity of underlying pulmonary disease
2. To estimate the risk of pulmonary complications
3. To optimize pulmonary function by correction of any reversible disease and minimize morbidity and mortality

### B. CLINICAL ASSESSMENT

1. History
   a. Dyspnea
      (1) Most common symptom indicative of pulmonary disease; requires evaluation of pulmonary function
      (2) Assessment made by determining degree of exertion that causes breathlessness.
      (3) Interpretation depends on patient's age, physical condition, and normal ventilatory capacity.
      (4) General evaluation obtained by questions directed toward ability to perform daily activities, such as walking, climbing stairs, carrying packages.
      (5) Acceptable cardiorespiratory function is suggested by absence of dyspnea after climbing two flights of stairs. Dyspnea on exertion can roughly be correlated with a reduction in forced expiratory volume in one second ($FEV_1$) to 50 per cent of predicted value.[1]
      (6) Dyspnea at rest indicates an advanced stage of lung (or cardiac) disease or, if new, an acute problem.
   b. Evaluate additional symptoms indicative of pulmonary

disease. Pain, especially if pleuritic, must be evaluated for possible disease of the pleural or chest wall. Cough or hemoptysis may be indicative of pulmonary infection, tuberculosis, bronchogenic carcinoma, pulmonary infarct, or such cardiac problems as congestive heart failure or mitral stenosis.

2. Physical examination
   a. Observe the breathing pattern. If the patient uses accessory muscles of respiration with intercostal muscle retraction and nasal flaring, he is already dependent on reserve mechanisms to maintain ventilation and may be at high risk for postoperative respiratory failure.
   b. Note the quality of breath sounds as well as the percussion note (dull, resonant, or hyperresonant) and such extraneous sounds as rales, rhonchi, and wheezes.
   c. Assess cardiac sounds, including murmurs and loudness of $P_2$. Check for evidence of cor pulmonale.
   d. Determine whether clubbing of the nails is indicative of underlying disease.
   e. Remember that hypoxemia and hypercapnia are difficult to judge clinically and that such signs as cyanosis may be unreliable.

3. Laboratory assessment
   a. Spirometry
      (1) Allows the physician to confirm pulmonary disease and determine the degree of physiologic impairment. Spirometry has been used for many years to help identify pulmonary risk factors.[2]
      (2) Spirometry results are expressed both in terms of volume and as a percentage of a subject's predicted value (lung volumes depend on age, sex, height, and weight). Values less than 70 per cent of that predicted are considered abnormal.
      (3) Important measurements (see Fig. 3–1)
          (a) Forced vital capacity (FVC): Maximal inspiration to total lung capacity, followed by full expiration to residual volume, measured in liters
          (b) Forced expiratory volume in one second ($FEV_1$): A measure of airway resistance, provided maximal effort has been made
          (c) Typical changes in various types of lung diseases compared with normal are noted in Table 3–1.

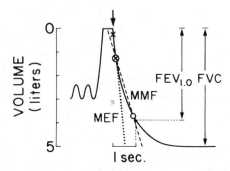

**Figure 3–1.** Analysis of forced expiratory spirogram for maximal expiratory flow (MEF, slope of line joining points at 200 ml and 1200 ml after start of expiration) and of maximal mid-expiratory flow (MMF, slope of a line joining points at 25 per cent and 75 per cent of FVC). Arrow indicates start of forced expiration.

    (d) Maximal breathing capacity (MBC): This parameter may be the single best predictor of postoperative complications, as noted by Gaensler.[3] It may be more useful than vital capacity or $FEV_1/FVC$, since the patient's ability to perform the test reflects many factors—presence of airway obstruction, mental status, muscle strength, and pain.

    (e) Additional useful parameters can be obtained from the forced expirogram.

        *1.* Maximal expiratory flow (MEF) is determined by measuring the slope of a line joining points at 200 ml and 1200 ml after

**TABLE 3–1. Lung Volume Assessment**

| Type of Dyspnea | FVC | $FEV_1$ | $FEV_1/FVC$ |
|---|---|---|---|
| Purely obstructive | Normal or slightly reduced | Reduced | Reduced (< 60%) |
| Purely restrictive | Reduced | Reduced proportionally or less to FVC | Normal or supernormal |
| Mixed | Reduced | Reduced | Reduced |

the start of expiration. This value reflects total respiratory resistance but depends on the amount of effort exerted by the patient. It can be useful in determining whether maximal effort has been made.

2. Maximal midexpiratory flow (MMF) is determined by measuring the slope of a line joining points at 25 per cent and 75 per cent of FVC. It is mostly effort-independent and is sensitive in detecting small-airway disease.

(f) More sophisticated tests of pulmonary mechanics, including flow-volume curves, closing volumes, and diffusion parameters, may be performed, but the studies mentioned earlier will suffice in most situations. Most likely pulmonary consultation will be required in more complex or in borderline situations.

b. Arterial blood gases

(1) Preoperative arterial blood gases should be obtained if respiratory impairment is suggested by the clinical history, the physical examination, or by pulmonary function tests.

(2) Hypoxemia

(a) $P_aO_2$ (arterial $PO_2$) is normally about 90 mm Hg in the young; it decreases progressively with age owing to ventilation-perfusion mismatching and may drop to the 70 mm Hg range by age 70.

(b) Hypoxemia has four main etiologies:

1. Aveolar hypoventilation

a. Carbon dioxide retention is the sine qua non.

b. Hypoxemia secondary to alveolar hypoventilation and carbon dioxide retention alone is uncommon preoperatively unless ventilation has been reduced by heavy sedation, trauma, or thoracic cage abnormalities. Postoperatively, sedative drugs, narcotics, incisional pain, casts, surgical dressing, etc. may result in relatively pure hypoventilation.

2. Ventilation-perfusion mismatch

a. Adequate gas exchange depends on matching the amount of blood perfusing the lung with the alveolar ventilation.

Because cardiac output is in the range of 5 liters/min and total alveolar ventilation is also about 5 liters/min, the ratio is close to one in a healthy person.

b. Various lung diseases can result in ventilation-perfusion mismatching owing to areas of the lung that are underventilated compared with perfusion (low $\dot{V}/\dot{Q}$ = shunting), or underperfused compared with ventilation (high $\dot{V}/\dot{Q}$ = dead space).

c. $\dot{V}/\dot{Q}$ abnormalities are the most common cause of arterial hypoxemia.

3. Diffusion defect

   a. Impaired diffusion of oxygen from the alveolus to the blood results from either loss of alveolar-capillary surface area for gas exchange (as in emphysema) or an interstitial process increasing the diffusion distance (as in pulmonary fibrosis).

   b. Hypoxemia at rest rarely results from a pure diffusion defect and is most often seen in combination with a $\dot{V}/\dot{Q}$ mismatch.

   c. $P_aCO_2$ is normal, since this gas is more diffusible.

4. Arteriovenous shunting

   a. Right-to-left shunting is an extreme degree of $\dot{V}/\dot{Q}$ abnormality—continued blood flow but no ventilation.

   b. Intrapulmonary arteriovenous shunting occurs most frequently with pneumonias, atelectasis, and shock lung.

(c) One hundred per cent oxygen will raise $P_aO_2$ to levels equal to those of a healthy person breathing 100 per cent oxygen if the hypoxemia is due either to ventilation-perfusion mismatch or to diffusion defects. However, 100 per cent oxygen will not correct a complete arteriovenous shunt and can be used to differentiate between these abnormalities.

(d) The alveolar–arterial oxygen pressure difference—the $P_{A-a}O_2$ gradient—is an important concept in determining whether arterial hypoxemia results from alveolar hypoventilation alone or from inefficient oxygen exchange due to $\dot{V}/\dot{Q}$ abnormality, shunting, or diffusion defect.

$$P_{A-a}O_2 \text{ gradient} = P_AO_2 - P_aO_2$$

where $P_AO_2 = (PB - PH_2O)(F_IO_2) - \dfrac{P_aCO_2}{R}$

where $P_AO_2$ = alveolar oxygen pressure
$P_aO_2$ = measured arterial oxygen pressure
PB = barometric pressure (at sea level = 760 mm Hg)
$PH_2O$ = partial pressure of $H_2O$ = 47 mm Hg
$F_IO_2$ = Fraction of inspired oxygen in inspired gas (21 per cent in room air)
R = respiratory quotient, assumed to be 0.8 in most instances

at room air

$$P_AO_2 = (760 - 47)(0.21) - \dfrac{P_aCO_2}{0.8}$$

$$= 150 - \dfrac{P_aCO_2}{0.8}$$

Taking the example of a healthy person and assuming a $P_aCO_2$ of 40,

$$P_AO_2 = 150 - \dfrac{40}{0.8} = 100$$

Since normal $P_aO_2$ (measured arterial oxygen) is about 90, the normal $P_{A-a}O_2$ gradient = $100 - 90 = 10$ mm Hg.

This normal 10 mm Hg gradient is due to a small degree of $\dot{V}/\dot{Q}$ mismatch in the normal lung. The $P_{A-a}O_2$ gradient remains normal in hypoxemia resulting from pure alveolar hypoventilation (normal lungs). It increases substantially over the normal 5 to 10 mm Hg in hypoxemia secondary to $\dot{V}/\dot{Q}$ mismatch or diffusion defects.

    (3) Hypercapnia

        (a) Hypercapnia should be recognized preoperatively because it generally indicates respiratory impairment and thus is implicated in increased surgical risk.

        (b) It is important to determine whether elevation of $P_aCO_2$ is acute or chronic. This judgment is based on the history, the physical examination, the evaluation of acid–base status, and the detection of easily correctable etiologies.

            *(1)* Acute and often correctable causes of ele-

vated $P_aCO_2$ include bronchospasm, laryngospasm, drugs (narcotics, sedatives), severe pneumonia or pulmonary edema, and pneumothorax.

(2) Chronic causes of elevated $P_aCO_2$ include chronic obstructive and severe restrictive lung disease, myopathy involving respiratory muscles, and CNS impairment.

c. Chest x-ray

   (1) A great deal of controversy exists over the need for preoperative chest x-rays.

   (2) In a recent study reported in *Lancet* that involved 10,000 consecutive non-cardiopulmonary surgery admissions, marked differences in preoperative utilization of chest x-rays were noted. There was no significant correlation with operative or anesthesia decisions nor with clinical outcome.[4]

   (3) In patients under age 30 significant abnormalities are rare, particularly if clinical suspicion is low.[5]

   (4) In terms of prescreening for lung cancer, routine x-rays are indicated in smokers, in people with chronic cough or bronchitis, and in men over age 60.[6]

   (5) Based on these and other findings from the literature, preoperative chest x-rays can be recommended in any of the following situations:

      (a) Cardiopulmonary abnormalities are suggested by history or physical examination

      (b) Patient is over age 40 (controversial if patient is asymptomatic)

      (c) Thoracic surgical procedure is scheduled

d. Electrocardiography

   (1) Indications for ECG are controversial.

   (2) ECG findings, such as right axis shift, right bundle-branch block, or right ventricular hypertrophy, may suggest more severe pulmonary disease than might be suspected by the history, physical examination, and chest x-ray.

   (3) Although there is no consensus, preoperative ECGs are reasonable in the following circumstances:

      (a) History or physical findings suggestive of cardiopulmonary disease

      (b) Thoracic or abdominal procedure is planned

      (c) As a baseline for comparison in patient over age 40

## C. CANDIDATES FOR PREOPERATIVE EVALUATION

1. Identification of patients by way of history, physical examination, chest x-ray, and ECG.
2. All patients in the following categories are considered to be at increased risk and should have preoperative pulmonary evaluations:
   a. Patients scheduled for thoracic surgery[7, 8]
   b. Patients undergoing upper abdominal surgery[9]
   c. Patients with history of cough and heavy smoking[10]
   d. Obese patients[11]
   e. Patients age 70 or older[12]
   f. Patients with pulmonary disease[13]

# II. ANALYSIS OF RISK FACTORS

## A. NON-PULMONARY RISK FACTORS

1. Smoking
   a. The incidence of postoperative complications is higher among smokers than among nonsmokers,[10] with the relative risk estimated to be two to six times greater in smokers.
   b. It may be that symptoms of respiratory tract disease, such as cough and dyspnea, accompanied by abnormal pulmonary function tests, are the determinants of increased risk rather than cigarette smoking per se.[10, 14]
2. Obesity
   a. Obesity has been associated with an increased risk of postoperative pulmonary complications, although the exact definition of obesity is variable:[11, 15] Body weight that is more than 30 per cent above ideal weight is a commonly accepted rule of thumb.
   b. Physiologic changes that accompany obesity include:
      (1) Decreasing functional residual capacity and expiratory reserve volume with increasing weight
      (2) Expiratory reserve volume smaller than closing volume, resulting in airway closure and an increase in the $P_{A-a}O_2$ gradient
      (3) Increased mechanical work of breathing because of excessive fat
   c. These physiologic changes may result in ineffective cough, atelectasis, progressive hypoxemia, and infections.
3. Age
   a. Age may increase the risk of postoperative morbidity and mortality, possibly related to normal decline in

pulmonary function as reflected by reduced lung volumes, expiratory flow, elastic recoil, and $P_aO_2$.

   b. This increased risk may be significant only after age 70. One study, however, did not demonstrate increased pulmonary complication with advanced age when other variables were corrected for.[10]

4. Surgery-related factors

   a. Common factors in all types of surgery that lead to pulmonary complications include diminution of lung volumes secondary to anesthesia, supine position, pain with impairment of full inspiration, narcotics (which depress respiration), abdominal distention, and bandages.

   b. The type of surgery greatly affects the incidence of pulmonary complications, owing largely to effects on postoperative lung volumes, as demonstrated in Figure 3–2.

     (1) Non-abdominal, non-thoracic surgery: Risk is low and related to anesthesia risk.

     (2) Abdominal surgery: As seen in Figure 3–2, there is a marked drop in postoperative vital capacity, which then gradually reverts toward normal. In the immediate postoperative period, vital capacity after upper abdominal surgery may be as low as 25 per cent of preoperative values, and after lower

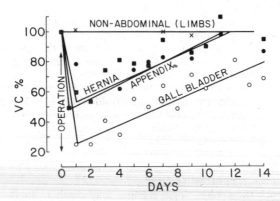

**Figure 3–2.** Change in vital capacity (VC, in per cent of preoperative value) following operations: gallbladder, ○; hernias, ●; appendectomies, ■; and nonabdominal (limbs), x. Adapted from Churchill ED, McNeil D: The reduction in vital capacity following operation. Surg. Gynecol Obstet *44*:483–488, 1927. By permission of Surgery, Gynecology and Obstetrics.

abdominal surgery, 50 per cent of preoperative values. The complication rate for upper abdominal surgery is predictably greater than that for lower abdominal surgery.

(3) Thoracic surgery: Vital capacity also falls postoperatively to about 50 per cent of preoperative values, but the complication rate also depends on the following:[16, 17]

    (a) Presence of chronic lung disease

    (b) Whether functional lung is resected

    (c) Amount of functional lung resected

    (d) Degree to which the bellows function of the lung is affected

5. Anesthesia-related factors

  a. Physiologic alterations during surgery

    (1) Progressive decrease in functional residual capacity owing to:

      (a) Cephalad shift in diaphragm in supine position caused by displacement of abdominal contents

      (b) Areas of microatelectasis and gas trapping

    (2) Alteration in ventilation-perfusion with positive pressure ventilation

      (a) Nondependent parts of the lung are relatively hyperventilated and underperfused ($\uparrow$ V/Q = dead space).

      (b) Dependent parts of the lung are hypoventilated and hyperperfused ($\downarrow$ V/Q = shunting), leading to hypoxemia.

      (c) Differs from normal awake subjects, or supine anesthetized subjects who are breathing spontaneously and who have both increased ventilation and perfusion in the dependent portions of the lung

    (3) Decreased mucosal clearance that promotes atelectasis by retention of secretions resulting from use of barbiturates, anesthetic agents and intubation, leading to increased risk of infection

  b. Duration of anesthesia

    (1) Regardless of other factors, an anesthesia time longer than three hours has been implicated in increased postoperative pulmonary complications.[17, 18]

  c. General vs. spinal anesthesia. Although spinal anesthesia itself does not suppress respiration, when it is used with sedation it can be more dangerous than general anesthesia with intubation, since the patient's airway and secretions are not controlled as well.[19]

6. Other non-pulmonary factors that may contribute to risk include general debilitation and malnutrition and acute respiratory infections.

## B. PULMONARY RISK FACTORS

1. Multiple studies have identified a number of pulmonary risk factors that place the patient at high risk for developing postoperative pulmonary complications (see Table 3–2).
2. Thoracic surgery
   a. Thoracic surgery adds another dimension to risk analysis, because lung tissue is resected. Resection may have one of three consequences:
      (1) Further impairment of lung function owing to removal of adjacent normal lung tissue
      (2) Little change in lung function (other than normal postoperative drop in vital capacity) after resection of nonfunctioning lung
      (3) Improvement in $P_aO_2$ owing to resection of lung with $\dot{V}/\dot{Q}$ imbalance, as noted earlier.
   b. Because of these variable effects of lung resection on pulmonary function, patients with marginal function require more specialized studies to determine whether they can tolerate lung resection and still maintain adequate postoperative pulmonary function. Currently available studies include:
      (1) Regional lung function using radionuclide scans
         (a) These split lung-function ventilation-perfusion studies provide a noninvasive method of assessing individual lung function and predicting postoperative vital capacity, $FEV_1$, and maximal breathing capacity.[21, 22]
      (2) Balloon occlusion of the pulmonary artery
         (a) Rarely, unilateral pulmonary artery occlusion is done in an effort to determine whether patients with severe pulmonary hypertension will have an adequate pulmonary vascular bed after resection.
   c. Total risk assessment must be based on a combination of the pulmonary and non-pulmonary risk factors already discussed. Because of the multiple contributing factors, precise predictions of risk are impossible, although an estimate of relative risk can be made. There are few absolute contradictions to surgery (except for limitations on lung resection), and potential benefits must be weighed against the risks of surgery or alternative treatment.

**TABLE 3–2. Pulmonary Tests Indicating High Risk of Morbidity and Mortality**

Spirometric studies
1. Maximal breathing capacity less than 50 per cent of predicted
2. Forced expiratory volume in one second less than 2 liters

Arterial blood gases
1. Arterial $Pco_2 > 45$ mm Hg
2. Hypoxemia – $P_aO_2 < 55$ mm Hg[20] – hypoxemia, however, may not be reliable in thoracic surgery, since an area of severe $\dot{V}/\dot{Q}$ imbalance (as in lung tumor) may be resected, which would improve postoperative $P_aO_2$.

Pulmonary vasculature
1. Pulmonary arterial pressure during temporary unilateral occlusion of left or right main pulmonary artery > 30 mm Hg.

Modified from Tisi GM: Preoperative evaluation of pulmonary function. Am Rev Respir Dis *119*:293–310, 1979.

## III. PROPHYLACTIC MEASURES THAT REDUCE PULMONARY RISK

**A.** As long ago as 1946, Dripps and Deming reported that among 1240 patients receiving general anesthesia, the incidence of postoperative atelectasis and pneumonia could be reduced from 11 per cent to 4 per cent "if a rational prophylactic regimen is observed prior to surgery, during operation, and immediately following operation."[23] Since that time a number of therapeutic maneuvers have been reported as being beneficial, including:[24]
  1. Preoperative cessation of ciagarette smoking
     a. As noted earlier, it is somewhat difficult to separate the operative risks that stem from underlying lung disease from those associated with smoking per se.
     b. In general, the patient should stop smoking for as long as possible before general anesthesia. Because it takes at least several weeks to see some improvement in airway clearance and reversal of small-airway disease, reports in the literature suggest that abstinence from smoking for at least two to four weeks may be required if significant differences in postoperative outcome are to be seen.[25]
     c. One immediate benefit of stopping cigarette smoking is reduction of carboxyhemoglobin levels in the blood, the half-life of carboxyhemoglobin while breathing room air being four hours. Oxygen delivery to tissue would therefore improve.

2. Antibiotic treatment of pulmonary infection
   a. Elective operations should be postoponed if a patient has an acute pulmonary infection, because patients with viral and bacterial bronchitis have some obstruction of the small airways, which increases the risks of postoperative atelectasis and pneumonia.
   b. If surgery cannot be postponed, pharmacologic treatment of bronchial or pulmonary infections of presumed bacterial etiology is justified.
3. Antibiotic treatment of chronic bronchitis
   a. Although the usefulness of prophylactic antibiotics is uncertain, some studies have suggested their utility, particularly in association with other measures.[26]
4. Preoperative psychologic preparation
   a. Preoperative orientation to the intensive care unit can reduce fear and increase cooperation. Preoperative preparation may also reduce pain and the need for narcotics and therefore the potential for respiratory depression.
5. Preoperative teaching of respiratory maneuvers
   a. Preoperative physical therapy instruction, including deep breathing exercises, has been shown to reduce the incidence of postoperative atelectasis more than when instructions are first given postoperatively.[28]
6. Preoperative bronchodilators for asthmatics[29]
   a. Maximal airway dilatation is essential in an effort to assist mucus clearance and prevent perioperative bronchospasm.
   b. Patients with a history of chronic cough, frequent respiratory tract infections, chronic obstructive pulmonary disease, wheezing, or asthma should be assessed for bronchospastic airway disease.
   c. Pulmonary function studies employing pre- and post-bronchodilator flow rates will give the most accurate information as to the usefulness of perioperative bronchodilators.
   d. Drugs
      (1) Theophylline derivatives generally are the choice for initial and maintenance therapy.
         (a) Theophylline levels between 10 and 20 $\mu g/$ml should be maintained. Levels above 20 $\mu g$ are associated with significant increases in toxicity.
         (b) For patients who have not taken any the-

ophylline preparations for 24 to 48 hours, a loading dose of 5 to 6 mg/kg is infused IV over 20 to 30 minutes, followed by a maintenance dose of 0.4 to 0.9 mg/kg/h.

1. The lower dosage must be used in patients with liver disease or congestive heart failure, in those who are over age 55, and in those who are using certain drugs (particularly cimetidine) owing to decreased metabolism of the bronchodilator.

2. Theophylline metabolism may be increased in smokers and in children under age 17, requiring possible increase in dosage.

(c) Patients already receiving a theophylline preparation should have their blood levels checked and dosage adjusted.

(d) If surgery is not emergent and the patient is not in distress, oral therapy may be started preoperatively with aminophylline, 3 to 6 mg/kg/q6h, or one of the many other theophylline preparations available.

(e) Because of the variations in absorption and metabolism, adequacy of dosage should be checked by determining blood levels of theophylline once a steady state has been reached.

(2) Oral therapy with beta$_2$-adrenergic agents may need to be added to the regimen if bronchospasm persists at maximal therapeutic theophylline levels. Terbutaline, 2.5 to 5 mg q6–8h; metaproterenol, 10 to 20 mg q6h; or albuterol, 2 to 4 mg q6–8h can be given.

7. Maintenance of good nutrition[29]

a. Nutritional status is an important consideration in every surgical patient, as debilitation may result in weakness of the respiratory muscles, apathy, and depressed ventilatory response to hypoxia. The catabolic state that exists postoperatively will further exacerbate any preoperative nutritional deficiency. Elective surgery should be delayed until nutritional support is optimized, as discussed elsewhere.

8. Minimization of duration of anesthesia

a. Patients whose anesthesia time exceeds three hours

are generally more likely to develop postoperative pulmonary complications.

9. Minimization of postoperative narcotic analgesia
   a. Narcotics suppress ventilation and may lead to increased pulmonary complications.
10. Maximization of inspiration
    a. The incentive spirometer has been shown to be the most effective method of preventing postoperative atelectasis and respiratory complications;[30] a sustained maximum inspiration is achieved and it is easy to use. Hourly usage is recommended, along with encouragement to cough and clear secretions. Blow bottles are variably effective, the main benefit being secondary to the maximal inspiration preceding forced expiration.
    b. Intermittent positive pressure breathing has not been found to have a beneficial effect in preventing postoperative atelectasis.
11. Early mobilization
    a. Because the upright position improves lung expansion and lung volumes compared with the supine position, early mobilization is important in reducing postoperative diminution in lung volumes.

## REFERENCES

1. Fenel V, Hansley MJ, Vandam LD: To Make the Patient Ready for Anesthesia. Menlo Park, Addison-Wesley, 1980, p 25.
2. Berath G, Crawford D: Function tests in pulmonary surgery. J Thorac Surg 22:414, 1951.
3. Gaensler EA, Cugell DW, Lingren I, et al: The role of pulmonary insufficiency in mortality and invalidism following surgery for pulmonary tuberculosis. J Thorac Surg 29:163, 1955.
4. Royal College of Radiologists: National study: Pre-operative chest radiology. Lancet 2:83, 1979.
5. Rees AM, Roberts CJ, Bligh AS, et al: Routine pre-operative chest radiography in non-cardiopulmonary surgery. Br Med J 1:1337, 1976.
6. Kubik A: Screening for lung cancer—high risk groups. Br Med J 2(7):666, 1970.
7. Mittman C: Assessment of operative risk in thoracic surgery. Am Rev Respir Dis 84:197, 1961.
8. Lockwood P: The principles of predicting risk of post-thoracotomy-function related complications in bronchogenic carcinoma. Respiration 30:329, 1973.
9. Diament ML, Palmer KNV: Post-operative changes in gas tensions of arterial blood and in ventilatory function. Lancet 2:180, 1966.
10. Latimer G, Dickman M, Clinton DW, et al: Ventilatory patterns and pulmonary complications after upper abdominal surgery

determined by preoperative and postoperative computerized spirometry and blood gas analysis. Am J Surg *122*:622, 1971.

11. Putnam H, Jenicek JA, Cellan CA, Wilson RD: Anesthesia in the morbidly obese. South Med J *67*:411, 1974.

12. Zeffren SE, Hartford CE: Comparative mortality for various surgical operations in older versus younger age groups. J Am Geriatr Soc *20*:485, 1972.

13. Stein M, Koota GM, Simon M, Frank H: Pulmonary evaluation of surgical patients. JAMA *181*:765, 1962.

14. Wightman JAK: A prospective survey of the incidence of postoperative pulmonary complications. Br J Surg *55*:85, 1968.

15. Strauss RJ, Wise L: Operative risks of obesity. Surg Gynecol Obstet *146*:286, 1978.

16. Tarhan S, Moffitt EA, Gessler AD, et al: Risk of anesthesia and surgery in patients with chronic bronchitis and chronic obstructive pulmonary disease. Surgery *74*:720, 1973.

17. Tisi GM: Preoperative evaluation of pulmonary function. Am Rev Respir Dis *119*:293, 1979.

18. Wightman JAK: A prospective survey of the incidence of postoperative pulmonary complications. Br J Surg *55*:85, 1968.

19. Hamilton WK, Sohall MD: Choice of anesthesia techniques in patients with acute pulmonary disease. JAMA *197*:789, 1977.

20. Hodgkin JD, Dines ED, Didier EP: Pre-operative evaluation of the patient with pulmonary disease. Mayo Clin Proc *48*:114, 1973.

21. Boysen PG, Block AJ, Olsen GN, et al: Prospective evaluation for pneumonectomy using the [99m]technetium quantitative perfusion lung scan. Chest *72*:422, 1977.

22. DeMeester TR, VanHeestum RL, Karas JR, et al: Preoperative evaluation with differential pulmonary function. Ann Thorac Surg *18*:61, 1974.

23. Dripps RD, Deming MVN: Postoperative atelectasis and pneumonia: Diagnosis, etiology, and management based upon 1240 cases of upper abdominal surgery. Ann Surg *94*:24, 1946.

24. Medical evaluation of the pre-operative patient. Med Clin North Am *63*:1294, 1979.

25. Wheatley IC, Hardy KJ, Barter CE: An evaluation of preoperative methods of preventing postoperative pulmonary complications. Anaesth Intensive Care *5*:56, 1977.

26. Stein M, Cassadra EL: Preoperative pulmonary evaluation and therapy for surgery patients. JAMA *211*:787, 1970.

27. Egbert LD, Bartlet GE, Welch CE, et al: Reduction of postoperative pain by encouragement and instruction of patients. N Engl J Med *270*:825, 1964.

28. Thoren L: Postoperative pulmonary complications: Observations on their prevention by means of physiotherapy. Acta Chir Scand *107*:193, 1954.

29. Williams CD, Brenowitz JB: Prohibitive lung function and major surgical procedures. Am J Surg *132*:763, 1976.

30. Iverson LIG, Echer RR, Fox HE, et al: A comparative study of IPPB, the incentive spirometer and blow bottles: The prevention of atelectasis following cardiac surgery. Ann Thorac Surg *25*:197, 1978.

# 4

## HEMATOLOGY

## I. HEMOSTATIC DISORDERS

### A. PREOPERATIVE EVALUATION

1. Purpose: To detect potential bleeding problems and minimize hemostatic dysfunction perioperatively
2. Clinical assessment
   a. History
      (1) A careful history is crucial because it may give the first indication of a potential hemostatic problem. Furthermore, certain bleeding conditions may be associated with normal routine laboratory studies, and more definitive studies might be considered only on the basis of high clinical suspicion, based on the history.
      (2) Should include questions concerning:
          (a) Unusual bleeding after prior surgery or dental procedures. A history of uncomplicated surgery suggests little likelihood of a silent bleeding diathesis.
          (b) Transfusion requirement after minor procedures
          (c) Easy bruising
          (d) Unexplained epistaxis, menorrhagia, or other cutaneous or mucous membrane bleeding
          (e) Unexplained hematuria or gastrointestinal tract bleeding
          (f) History of hematomas or hemarthrosis
          (g) Delayed bleeding after surgery or trauma
          (h) Family history of bleeding disorder
          (i) Drug history. A large number of drugs may adversely affect hemostasis through a wide range of mechanisms. A careful and complete medication history must be obtained and each drug evaluated for its possible effects.

b. Physical examination may yield clues to an underlying disorder.
  (1) Lymphadenopathy, hepatomegaly, splenomegaly: Signs suggestive of lymphoproliferative or other neoplastic disease, infectious disease, or collagen vascular disorder
  (2) Petechiae, ecchymoses: May indicate a quantitative or qualitative platelet disorder
  (3) Joint deformity: Possibly associated with coagulopathy
  (4) Telangiectasias: May be due to hereditary Osler-Weber-Rendu disease
c. Laboratory assessment
  (1) Routine preoperative screening tests for evaluation of hemostatic function should include complete blood count (CBC) with differential, prothrombin time (PT), activated partial thromboplastin time (APTT), platelet count, and possibly, a bleeding time (particularly if the patient is taking a platelet-inhibiting agent, e.g., aspirin).

## B. PLATELET DISORDERS AND RISKS FOR SURGERY

1. Quantitative abnormalities (thrombocytopenia)
  a. Risk of bleeding in thrombocytopenia is directly related to the platelet count. Bleeding time does not become prolonged until the platelet count is less than 100,000, after which there is a linear prolongation of bleeding time with decrease in platelets, as seen in Figure 4–1. Clinical bleeding is rare when the platelet count is greater than 50,000 to 60,000, although variations may occur that depend on surgical factors. Below a count of 20,000, bleeding complications are common.
  b. The four main etiologies for thrombocytopenia are as follows:
    (1) Decreased platelet production (secondary to aplastic anemia, bone marrow infiltration, drugs [e.g., thiazides, alcohol], radiation, or ineffective erythropoiesis secondary to vitamin deficiencies and refractory anemias)
    (2) Increased platelet destruction as a result of hypersplenism, DIC (disseminated intravascular coagulation), TTP (thrombotic thrombocytopenic purpura), prosthetic heart valves, extracorporeal circulation, or by way of immunologically mediated processes, resulting in anti-platelet antibod-

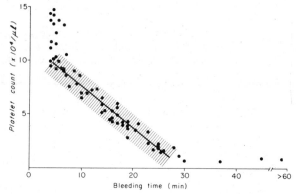

**Figure 4–1.** Effect of thrombocytopenia on bleeding time. (From Harker LA, Slichter ST: The bleeding time as a screening test for evaluation of platelet function. N Engl J Med *287*:156–159, 1972.)

ies caused by drug use, collagen disease, lympho-proliferative disease, and post-transfusion complications
  (3) Sequestration of platelets owing to an enlarged spleen (as seen in myeloproliferative disorders, infections, cirrhosis, Gaucher's disease, lympho-proliferative disorders, and sarcoidosis)
  (4) Dilution owing to massive blood transfusions
c. Perioperative management
  (1) Management should be directed toward either treatment and reversal of the underlying disease or elimination of external causative factors (e.g., drugs, radiation). If possible, surgery should be postponed until the condition is corrected or improved.
  (2) In emergency or refractory cases, patients should be transfused before surgery.
    (a) Sufficient platelets should be given to increase the preoperative count to 100,000/cu mm and maintained three to four days.
    (b) As a general rule, a single unit of random donor platelets will raise the count by about 5,000/cu mm. The half-life is about two to three days.
    (c) After transfusion the platelet increment should be checked at 1 hour and between 12 and 24 hours to ensure that there is good potential for recovery and survival.

     (d) Patients with increased platelet destruction will also rapidly destroy transfused platelets and may not adequately respond until the underlying disorder is controlled.

   (3) In massive transfusions, platelet concentrates should be given after 8 to 10 units of blood have been received. Moderate thrombocytopenia is common, since platelets survive only 72 hours at room temperature and stored blood contains few viable platelets.

   (4) After cardiopulmonary bypass, platelet counts routinely decrease to about 50 per cent of preoperative levels as a result of destruction in the perfusion apparatus, but this rarely in itself causes significant bleeding.

2. Qualitative abnormalities
   a. Qualitative platelet abnormalities may be acquired or hereditary. Bleeding time in the absence of thrombocytopenia is used as a screening test. If a qualitative defect is suspected, a hematology consultation is necessary so that aggregation studies may be performed.
   b. Acquired defects are most common and may result from the following:
      (1) Aspirin ingestion
         (a) Most common cause of qualitative abnormality
         (b) Has irreversible effect on platelet aggregation and thus may interfere with platelet function for 7 to 10 days.
         (c) Although aspirin increases bleeding time it is still generally within the normal four to nine minutes for most people and should not have clinical significance.
      (2) Ingestion of other drugs that affect platelet function
         (a) Nonsteroidal anti-inflammatory drugs have aspirinlike effects on platelets, with indomethacin and phenylbutazone being the most potent.
         (b) Many other drugs having less potent effects include dipyridamole, penicillin (high dose), carbenicillin, beta blockers, antidepressants, and ethanol. Each drug taken by the patient should be checked for possible effects on platelet function.
      (3) Systemic disorders, such as uremia, systemic lupus erythematosus, alcoholism, liver disease, myelo-

proliferative disorders, leukemia, and dysproteinemias

c. Hereditary qualitative platelet defects are uncommon and include the following:
   (1) Thrombasthenia, a disorder in which platelets have a normal release reaction but lack subsequent aggregation
   (2) Bernard–Soulier syndrome, in which platelet morphology is markedly abnormal
   (3) Other rare diseases, such as Wiskott-Aldrich syndrome, hereditary afibrinogenemia, mucopolysaccharidosis, cyanotic congenital heart disease, and glycogen storage disease
   (4) Von Willebrand's disease is characterized by abnormal platelet aggregation and adhesiveness resulting from disturbance of von Willebrand's factor, a plasma protein. In addition, factor VIII activity is low (this is discussed more fully later).
d. Perioperative management
   (1) In general, therapy should be directed at the underlying cause.
   (2) Aspirin and other drugs that affect platelets should be withheld for at least a week before surgery.
   (3) Transfusion of normal platelets for most qualitative disorders is efficacious. Exceptions include:
      (a) Uremia: In uremic patients with prolonged bleeding time, dialysis should be carried out immediately before surgery.
      (b) Von Willebrand's: Patients with this disorder require infusion of fresh frozen plasma or cryoprecipitate.
      (c) Dysproteinemias: Treat underlying disease.

3. Thrombocytosis
   a. Defined as platelet count above 350,000/cu mm.
   b. Associated conditions include malignancy, iron deficiency, chronic inflammatory diseases, and asplenia.
   c. Thrombotic or hemorrhagic manifestations usually occur with platelet counts greater than 1,000,000.
   d. Treatment is directed at the underlying disorder. If emergency therapy is required, plateletpheresis will rapidly reduce the quantity of circulating platelets. Alkylating agents and $^{32}$P will have slower onset of action.

## C. COAGULATION DISORDERS

1. Activated partial thromboplastin time measures the conversion of factor XII to fibrin (intrinsic pathway); factors

VIII, IX, XI, and XII are unique to APTT. Prothrombin time measures the rate of formation of fibrin in the presence of tissue factor (extrinsic pathway). Factor VII is required only in PT. Factors V, X, prothrombin, and fibrinogen are required for both PT and APTT.

2. Abnormal APTT *or* PT. An 80 per cent loss of coagulation factors is required to prolong PT and APTT.

a. Hereditary factor deficiencies

(1) Abnormal APTT, normal PT

(a) Most common: Factor VIII deficiency (hemophilia), factor IX deficiency (Christmas disease)

(b) Rarer: Factor XI and XII deficiencies. There is no tendency to bleed with factor XII deficiency (Hageman factor).

(c) Von Willebrand's: Autosomal dominant disorder, which may have few symptoms of bleeding diathesis before surgery, or may be associated with lifelong history of easy bruising, mucosal bleeding, and hemorrhage. Usually APTT and bleeding time are prolonged but may be normal (see explanation under 4a(2). The disorder is characterized by decrease in factor VIII antigen (VIII AGN), factor VIII coagulant activity (VIII AHF), and von Willebrand's factor (VIII VWF), which are required to support ristocetin aggregation of platelets.

(2) Abnormal PT, normal APTT: Factor VII deficiency

b. Acquired circulatory inhibitors of specific factors

(1) Most commonly seen in patients with severe hemophilia who receive frequent factor VII and develop immunoglobulin G antibodies

(2) Rarely, patients without factor deficiency syndromes may develop inhibitor, usually against factor VIII, in association with certain diseases, such as inflammatory bowel disease, collagen disease, penicillin reaction, and old age.

3. Abnormal APTT *and* PT. A number of etiologies exist, including:

a. Deficiency of factors II (prothrombin), V, or X. Dysfibrinogenemia may be associated with normal or prolonged studies.

b. Deficiency of more than one coagulation factor

c. Presence of inhibitor to one or more coagulation

factors. Patients with systemic lupus erythematosus may have a circulating anticoagulant that prolongs APTT and PT but does not cause significant bleeding.

d. Disseminated intravascular coagulation
e. Vitamin K deficiency secondary to:
    (1) Oral anticoagulants
    (2) Inadequate intake
    (3) Broad-spectrum antibiotics (suppress vitamin K–producing bacteria), particularly in association with reduced intake or debilitation
    (4) Malabsorption (pancreatic deficiency, small bowel, or biliary disease)
    (5) Liver parenchymal disease
        Generally, PT is affected more than APTT in vitamin K deficiency.

4. Abnormal bleeding tendency by history but normal coagulation studies and platelets. It must not be assumed that routine screening procedures eliminate the possibility of all hereditary or acquired coagulation disorders. A hematology consultation should always be obtained if an underlying bleeding diathesis is suspected.
    a. Special studies may be needed to rule out:
        (1) Factor XIII (fibrin stabilizing factor) deficiency. Suspected by history if good initial hemostasis follows surgery or trauma, but after one or two days bleeding starts again and continues. The urea clot solubility test must be performed for diagnosis.
        (2) Von Willebrand's (which may have normal routine screening tests). Factor VIII AGN and factor VIII VWF may be needed for diagnosis.
        (3) Dysfibrinogenemias. Fibrinogen levels and tests to determine dysfunctional fibrinogens may be necessary.
    b. Patient must be examined carefully for signs of other systemic diseases that may cause bleeding, to rule out:
        (1) Osler-Weber-Rendu: capillary telangiectasias
        (2) Ehlers-Danlos: hyperextensibility, tissue-paper scars
        (3) Vasculitis: purpuric rash
        (4) See Table 4–1 for summary.

5. Perioperative management
    a. Factor deficiency syndromes
        (1) Replacement therapy should be as specific as possible, with factor levels monitored closely with a ten-day to two-week course of therapy. See Table 4–2 for recommended protocols.

**TABLE 4–1. Coagulation Test Results in Hereditary Factor Deficiencies**

| Abnormal | Normal | Disorder |
|---|---|---|
| APTT | PT | Hemophilia (factor VIII); Christmas disease (factor IX); factors XI, XII (Hageman); von Willebrand's |
| PT | APTT | Factor VII |
| APTT, PT | | Factors II (prothrombin), V, X; dysfibrinogenemias; deficiency of or inhibitor to one or more coagulation factors, DIC, vitamin K deficiency, broad-spectrum antibiotics, malabsorption, liver disease |
| | PT, APTT | Factor XIII (fibrin stabilizing factor), von Willebrand's, dysfibrinogenemias, Osler-Weber-Rendu, Ehlers-Danlos, vasculitis |

**TABLE 4–2. Protocol for Replacement of Coagulation Factors**

| Factor | Percent of Normal Required | | Material | Dose per Kg | Repeat (hr) |
|---|---|---|---|---|---|
| | MINOR SURGERY | MAJOR SURGERY | | | |
| I (fibrinogen) | 20 | 40 | Cryoprecipitate | 0.3 bag | 48 |
| II (pro-thrombin) | 40 | 40 | Plasma | 20 ml | 24 |
| V | 10 | 15 | Plasma | 10 ml | 12 |
| VII | 10 | 20 | Plasma | 10 ml | 6 |
| VIII | 40 | 80 | Concentrate[a"] | 40 units | 6[b] |
| IX | 40 | 80 | Concentrate[c] | 80 units | 6[d] |
| X | 15 | 20 | Plasma | 10 ml | 24 |
| XI | ? | ?30 | Plasma | 20 ml | 48 |
| XII | ? | ? | None | None | |
| XIII | 5 | 5 | Cryoprecipitate or Plasma | 0.1 bag 5 ml | 48 48 |
| VWF | 50 | ? | Cryoprecipitate | 0.6 bag | 8 |

[a] or cryoprecipitate
[b] or better given 5 units per kg per hour
[c] or plasma
[d] dose—40 units per kg or preferably 5 units per kg per hour
From Watson-Williams EJ: Medical evaluation of the preoperative patient. Med Clin North Am *63*:1183, 1979.

   b. Treatment of circulatory inhibitors
      (1) Treatment must be individualized. Some patients may need no treatment (some lupus inhibitors, as noted earlier), whereas others may need large quantities of the coagulation factor to overcome the inhibitor, or cytotoxic therapy to suppress the inhibitor. Hematology consultation is necessary for these complex cases.
   c. Anticoagulants
      (1) Coumarin anticoagulants
         (a) Interfere with action of vitamin K in synthesis of factors II, VII, IX, X
         (b) Discontinuation of coumarin results in normalization of PT within 36 to 48 hours.
         (c) Vitamin K given IV (10 to 15 mg) can correct PT within 8 to 12 hours but must be given with caution because of the possibility of anaphylaxis. Vitamin K may be given IM (not recommended because local hematoma formulation is possible), subcuataneously, or orally. It may be variably absorbed orally, and correction of PT may take longer (18 to 24 hours).
         (d) It is preferable simply to discontinue coumarin and not give vitamin K if possible, since a single dose may interfere with subsequent postoperative anticoagulants for as long as a week.
         (e) Emergency surgery may be performed by discontinuing coumarin and transfusing 2 to 4 units of fresh frozen plasma. This procedure may need to be repeated postoperatively.
      (2) Heparin
         (a) Coagulation as measured by APTT will be normal if heparin is discontinued eight hours before surgery.
         (b) Rapid reversal may be achieved by giving protamine sulfate, which neutralizes heparin milligram per milligram. The usual dose is about 50 mg of protamine administered IV over five minutes.
         (c) Although prolongation of the APTT, resulting in hemorrhage, is the most common complication of heparin therapy, heparin-induced thrombocytopenia is more common than generally recognized.[1] A platelet count before

heparinization is mandatory; if thrombocytopenia does occur, the heparin must be neu-
tralized with protamine sulfate before platelet
transfusion.

# II. ANEMIA

## A. PREOPERATIVE EVALUATION

1. Purpose
   a. To determine the level of hemoglobin and hematocrit
      required to provide adequate tissue oxygenation for
      the individual patient undergoing surgery
   b. To detect an underlying disorder that might result in
      further hematologic compromise in the perioperative
      period
2. Clinical assessment
   a. History
      (1) Should include questions regarding:
          (a) Diet
          (b) Previous use of hematinics (e.g., iron, folate)
          (c) Medications, particularly aspirin
          (d) Alcohol
          (e) Prior transfusions
          (f) Associated chronic illnesses
          (g) Family history of anemia or blood disorders
      (2) Assessment of severity of symptoms related to
          the anemia that may give a clue as to whether
          the patient's condition is acute or chronic, such
          as chest pain, shortness of breath, dizziness
   b. Physical examination. Clues might be found by eval-
      uating for:
      (1) Lymphadenopathy
      (2) Hepatosplenomegaly
      (3) Petechiae
      (4) Pallor
      (5) Hematest of stools
      (6) Evidence of chronic disease (e.g., liver, collagen
          vascular)
   c. Laboratory assessment
      Routine studies should include hemoglobin, he-
      matocrit, and red cell indices. If the results of any of
      these studies are abnormal, valuable information can
      be obtained from the blood smear, reticulocyte count,
      and Coombs' test, which will help evaluation of the
      etiology by classifying the disorder on the basis of red

cell morphology. Once the differential diagnosis has been narrowed, bone marrow examination and more specific studies might be indicated.

## B. NORMOCHROMIC–NORMOCYTIC ANEMIA

1. Increased reticulocytes
   a. Blood loss (several days)
   b. Hemolysis
      (1) Coombs' test positive
         (a) Autoimmune
            *(1)* Drug related (e.g., methyldopa)
            *(2)* Systemic disease (collagen vascular, malignancy)
            *(3)* Idiopathic
         (b) Isoimmune
            *(1)* Transfusion reaction
            *(2)* Newborn
      (2) Coombs' test negative
         (a) Increased red-cell fragility
            *(1)* Hereditary spherocytosis
            *(2)* Hereditary elliptocytosis
         (b) Decreased red-cell fragility: abnormal hemoglobins
         (c) Normal red-cell fragility
            *(1)* Alcohol
            *(2)* Toxins (drug, exotoxins)
            *(3)* Enzyme deficiencies (G6PD)
            *(4)* Lead poisoning
            *(5)* Vasculitis and microangiopathy
            *(6)* Hypersplenism
2. Decreased reticulocytes
   a. Hypoplastic anemia
   b. Chronic disease
   c. Endocrine deficiency
   d. Leukemias
3. Normal reticulocytes
   a. Acute blood loss
   b. Chronic renal disease

## C. HYPOCHROMIC, MICROCYTIC ANEMIA

1. Iron deficiency ($\downarrow$ Fe, $\uparrow$ Total iron-binding capacity [TIBC], less than 15 per cent saturation)
   a. Bleeding most common cause (e.g., peptic ulcer disease, gastritis, polyps, carcinoma, parasites, such medications as aspirin and nonsteroidal anti-inflammatory drugs)

2. Anemia of chronic disease ( $\downarrow$ Fe, $\downarrow$ TIBC, greater than 15 per cent saturation, ferritin normal or $\uparrow$ )
3. Sideroblastic anemia ( $\uparrow$ Fe, normal TIBC, greater than 60 per cent saturation, ferritin normal or $\uparrow$ )
4. Thalassemia minor (normal to $\uparrow$ Fe, normal TIBC, greater than 15 per cent saturation, ferritin normal or $\uparrow$ )

## D. MACROCYTIC ANEMIA

1. Megaloblastic
   a. Folate deficiency secondary to diet, malabsorption, drugs (phenytoin), pregnancy
   b. $B_{12}$ deficiency (pernicious anemia, ileal disease)
2. Liver disease
3. Hypothyroidism
4. Elevated reticulocytes

## E. PERIOPERATIVE MANAGEMENT AND SURGICAL RISKS

1. The discovery of anemia preoperatively is always a source for concern. How much of the evaluation can be deferred must be individualized on the basis of the history, physical examination, and laboratory findings, but there is little excuse to proceed with an elective procedure before evaluating the etiology of the anemia. Diagnosing iron deficiency before surgery is critical to raise the suspicion of a source of blood loss, usually from the gastrointestinal tract. Subsequent identification and treatment may prevent hemorrhagic perioperative complications. Although a complete discussion of every type of anemia and its treatment is beyond the scope of this manual, an understanding of general principles of evaluation and treatment is important. Except for emergency procedures, the source of anemia should be identified and treatment individualized on the basis of etiology when possible.
2. Hemoglobin requirements
   a. A hemoglobin of 9 to 10 gm/dl and hematocrit of 30 per cent have customarily been required to assure that tissue oxygenation is adequate during surgery.[2] The ideal balance between reduced oxygen transport caused by low hematocrit and increased viscosity from a high hematocrit has been variously reported between hematocrits of 30 per cent and 42 per cent.[2, 3]
   b. Although a hemoglobin of 10 gm/dl and a hematocrit of 30 per cent are general guidelines for acceptable preoperative values, each patient's requirement must

be assessed based on several factors, and a decision for transfusion must be made weighing the benefits of transfusion versus the risks.

(1) Factors requiring higher preoperative hemoglobin levels
   (a) Old age
   (b) Acute blood loss
   (c) Coronary artery disease
   (e) Pulmonary disease
   (f) Cerebrovascular or peripheral vascular disease
   (g) Significant anticipated loss of blood

(2) Factors making lower preoperative hemoglobin levels more acceptable
   (a) Youth
   (b) Chronic anemia
   (c) Normal exercise tolerance
   (d) No cardiac, pulmonary, or cerebrovascular disease
   (e) Little anticipated loss of blood

3. Therapy
   a. If perioperative red blood cell transfusion is required, therapy should provide only those blood components required to correct the defect. For purely elective surgery, treatment with oral replacement therapy (iron folate, $B_{12}$) is appropriate if surgery can wait.
   b. Packed red blood cells can be used for all but severe hemorrhage. Advantages over whole blood include reduced potassium and citrate load (which can complex with and lower $Ca^{++}$) and reduced risk of allergic response or reaction to antibodies in donor plasma.
   c. Transfusion reactions
      (1) Immediate or rapid onset due to:
         (a) Hemolysis of transfused RBCs
         (b) Allergic reaction to transfused RBCs, leukocytes, platelet antigens
         (c) Allergic reaction to plasma
         (d) Contamination of blood products by bacteria
      (2) Symptoms include fever, chills, nausea, vomiting, back pain, dyspnea, tachycardia, chest pain, edema, urticaria, and shock.
      (3) If transfusion reaction is suspected:
         (a) Stop transfusion immediately.
         (b) Repeat blood typing and cross-matching and perform Coombs' test on patient's cells.
         (c) Test serum of donor and patient for blood group antibodies

   (d) If sepsis is suspected, obtain blood cultures.
   (e) Check blood and urine for free hemoglobin, which would indicate hemolysis.
(4) Patients who develop febrile transfusion reactions without hemolysis may be sensitized to antigens on leukocytes or platelets. Transfusion should be done with washed RBCs, which have a lower content of these products and carry a lower risk for hepatitis.
(5) Autologous blood can be collected before an elective procedure and stored.
(6) Massive transfusion can be complicated by dilutions of platelets and coagulation factors and can lower the ionized $CA^{++}$ owing to complex formation with citrate. Platelet concentrates, fresh frozen plasma, and cryoprecipitate may be given after 10 to 12 units of RBCs, or fresh whole blood may be used every fourth unit. Slow infusion of 10 ml of 10% calcium gluconate every 4 or 5 units will prevent hypocalcemia.
(7) Transmission of communicable agents is the primary long-term risk of transfusions. Non-A, non-B hepatitis accounts for the majority of transfusion-related disease, but hepatitis B, cytomegalovirus, or toxoplasmosis may also occur. Concern recently has been raised about the possible transmission of acquired immune deficiency syndrome through blood products.

## III. ERYTHROCYTOSIS

A. Important to recognize preoperatively, as erythrocytosis may increase blood viscosity significantly (particularly above hematocrits of 55 per cent), resulting in circulatory stasis. One study shows cerebral blood flow is 50 per cent greater with a hematocrit between 36 per cent and 46 per cent than between 47 per cent and 53 per cent.[4]

## B. ETIOLOGIES

1. Stress erythrocytosis (Gaisböck's syndrome)
   a. Caused by decreased plasma volume, not increased red cell mass
   b. Patient is usually hypertensive, high-strung, and overweight
   c. Control of hypertension often restores plasma volume and hematocrit to normal

2. True erythrocytosis
   a. Primary (polycythemia rubra vera; see *Myeloprolifer-ative Disorders* below)
   b. Secondary
      (1) Tissue hypoxia
          (a) Chronic obstructive pulmonary disease
          (b) Cardiovascular anomalies with right-to-left shunt
          (c) High altitude
          (d) Hemoglobinopathy with increased oxygen affinity
      (2) Renal disease
          (a) Polycystic disease
          (b) Hydronephrosis
          (c) Bartter's syndrome
          (d) Transplant
      (3) Tumors
          (a) Renal cell carcinoma
          (b) Hepatoma
          (c) Adrenal tumors
          (d) Cerebellar hemangioblastoma
          (e) Uterine fibroids
   c. Treatment of true erythrocytosis depends on treatment of the underlying etiology when possible.

## IV. NEUTROPENIA

### A. ETIOLOGIES

1. Drugs (e.g., antineoplastic agents, antimicrobial agents, sulfonamides, chloramphenicol, antithyroid agents, propylthiouracil)
2. Infectious agent, particularly viral
3. Pre-leukemia, myeloproliferative disorders, and defects in myeloid maturation
4. Congenital
5. Chronic rheumatoid disease (systemic lupus erythematosus, Felty's syndrome)

### B. PERIOPERATIVE MANAGEMENT

1. Cancellation of surgery for count less than 1000/cu mm; risk of infection markedly increased when granulocyte count is less than 500/cu mm.
2. Treatment of underlying etiology; postponement of surgery in viral or drug-induced cases until leukopenia is reversed

3. Emergency surgery should be limited to diversion and drainage procedures
4. Granulocyte transfusions have little indication for surgery and only in an infected patient with a count less than 500/cu mm.

# V. SPECIAL HEMATOLOGIC CONSIDERATIONS

## A. LIVER DISEASE

1. Increased risk of bleeding owing to several etiologies
   a. Reduced synthesis of coagulation factors II, V, VII, IX, X, and possibly, XI and XII
   b. Related biliary tract disease with reduced level of bile salts and decreased absorption of fat-soluble vitamin K
   c. Increased risk of DIC, owing to reduced clearance of activated coagulation proteins
   d. Thrombocytopenia secondary to hypersplenism, marrow suppression, folate deficiency
   e. Bleeding from varices, ulcer, gastritis
2. Treatment
   a. Elimination of offending agents, particularly ethanol (ETOH)
   b. Coagulation factor abnormalities may not be corrected with vitamin K in severe liver disease. Fresh frozen plasma will transiently provide coagulation factors, and 2 to 4 units should be given preoperatively if coagulation abnormalities are not corrected by vitamin K. Risk of bleeding may require additional fresh frozen plasma postoperatively (or whole blood, if patient is actively bleeding).
   c. Transfused platelets may be ineffective if hypersplenism is the etiology for thrombocytopenia.

## B. SICKLE CELL DISEASE

1. Complications
   a. High risk of vaso-occlusive events in the perioperative period
   b. Other risk factors owing to sickling include severe anemia, cardiac and pulmonary disease, cholelithiasis, and susceptibility to infection, hypoxia, dehydration, and acidosis.
   c. Vaso-occlusive crisis may be difficult to differentiate from an acute abdomen.

2. Treatment
   a. Aggressive hydration, oxygenation, and alkalization to minimize factors initiating or exacerbating the sickle crises
   b. Exchange transfusion
      (1) Goal is to reduce potentially sickling cells to less than 30 per cent of total RBCs as checked by quantitative hemoglobin electrophoresis.
      (2) For elective procedures, gradual removal of 1 to 2 units of whole blood from the patient and replacement with 2 to 4 units of packed cells at a time may be started several weeks before surgery in an effort to raise the hemoglobin to a range of 12 to 13 gm/dl. Emergency surgery may necessitate more rapid exchange.

C. **MYELOPROLIFERATIVE DISORDERS (polycythemia vera, chronic myelogenous leukemia, myeloid metaplasia, essential thrombocythemia)**
   1. Increased surgical risk due to a variety of complications
      a. Polycythemia vera with increased red cell mass results in stasis, impaired blood flow, and tissue hypoxia. Thrombocytosis and qualitative platelet disorders cause thrombotic and bleeding complications. One study found a greater than 90 per cent risk of thrombotic or hemorrhagic complication, with a 36 per cent death rate in patients undergoing surgery with uncontrolled polycythemia vera. Preoperative control reduced the complication rate to 28 per cent with 5 per cent mortality, and long-term control resulted in little risk.[5]
      b. Uncontrolled leukocytosis may also result in tissue hypoxia secondary to leukostasis.
      c. Increased infection risk in patients with leukopenia, particularly with granulocyte count below 500/cu mm
   2. Treatment
      a. Red cell mass, platelet count, and white blood cells should be controlled by chemotherapy before elective surgery.
      b. In polycythemia, hematocrit should be reduced to about 45 per cent by phlebotomy.
      c. Platelet counts should be reduced below 1 million, but bleeding episode can occur owing to thrombocytopathy in the myeloproliferative disorders.
      d. White blood cell counts should be reduced to less than 50,000 before surgery. With counts greater than

100,000, leukapheresis should be performed for emergency surgery.

## D. DYSPROTEINEMIAS

1. Complications
   a. Abnormal quantities of immunoglobulins can alter blood viscosity, resulting in bleeding from mucous membranes and oozing after surgery. This is most commonly seen in Waldenström's macroglobulinemia but may also occur in about 10 per cent of patients with multiple myeloma owing to IgG.
   b. Immunoglobulins may also coat platelets, resulting in interference with adhesiveness and aggregation, which in turn results in prolongation of bleeding time.
   c. Hypercalcemia (particularly in multiple myeloma), infection, and impaired renal function are additional complications.
2. Perioperative management
   a. Plasmapheresis should be done in patients with increased viscosity greater than 4 (1.4 to 1.8 is normal).
   b. Bleeding time and platelet function should be studied preoperatively.
   c. Increase fluid intake to prevent dehydration.
   d. Control hypercalcemia, if present, by hydration, steroids, or mithramycin, if needed.

## VI. THROMBOEMBOLIC DISEASE

**A.** The risk of thromboembolic disease must be considered in every preoperative evaluation, because development of deep vein thrombosis in postoperative patients is extremely high (see Table 4–3). The prevalence of fatal pulmonary emboli in general surgery patients over age 40 approaches 1 per cent and in hip fractures, as high as 7 per cent.

**B.** Risk factors for development of thrombotic complications of deep vein thrombosis and pulmonary emboli include venous disease, prolonged immobilization, obesity, congestive heart failure, certain types of surgery (orthopaedic, prostatic, gynecologic), cancer, some hematologic disorders (e.g., polycythemia vera), and age.

## C. LOW-DOSE HEPARIN PROPHYLAXIS

1. Multiple studies have supported the safety and efficiency of low-dose subcutaneous heparin prophylaxis in reduc-

TABLE 4–3. Occurrence of Fatal Pulmonary Emboli in Surgical Patients

| Type of Surgery | Prevalence (%) |
| --- | --- |
| General | |
| Age >40 | 16–42 |
| Age >60 | 46–61 |
| Malignancy | 40–59 |
| Major gynecologic | 26 |
| With malignant disease | 35 |
| Without malignant disease | 10 |
| Urologic | |
| Open prostatectomy | 28–42 |
| Transurethral resection | 10 |
| Other | 31–58 |
| Thoracic | 12–26 |
| Neurosurgery | |
| Craniotomy | 18–40 |
| Laminectomy | 4–25 |
| Orthopaedic | |
| Total hip replacement | 40–78 |
| Hip fracture | 48–75 |
| Tibial fracture | 45 |
| Knee surgery | 57 |

From Rose SD: Prophylaxis of thromboembolic disease, in Medical evaluation of the preoperative patient. Med Clin North Am 63:1205–1225, 1979.

ing the incidence of fatal pulmonary emboli in general surgical patients, including the largest study of more than 4000 patients in a multicentered trial.[6]

2. Recommended treatment consists of administering 5000 units of heparin subcutaneously at least two hours before surgery, and then 5000 units every 12 hours after surgery for the duration of hospitalization. Double-blind studies do not show an increased risk of bleeding.

3. Exclusions to the use of low-dose heparin
   a. Orthopaedic surgery
      (1) Orthopaedic patients with fractures of the lower extremity or the hip, as well as patients undergoing surgery on these areas seem to receive little, if any, benefit from low-dose heparin prophylaxis based on multiple studies.[7, 8] However, a recent study by Leyvraz and co-workers[9] provides evidence that one can reduce the incidence of thrombosis significantly after hip replacement by ad-

justing the dose of prophylactic subcutaneous heparin to yield APTT in the high normal range, thereby restoring normal hemostatic equilibrium.
(2) In at least one study aspirin has been shown to decrease postoperative deep vein thrombosis in men undergoing orthopedic procedures, but not in women.[10]
  b. Prostate surgery: The usefulness of prophylactic heparin in open prostatectomy is still controversial; however, it does seem to be effective in other urologic procedures.

**D.** Physical measures, such as the following, should be used to reduce the risk of thromboembolic disease in patients who are not candidates for low-dose heparin.
  1. External pneumatic compression, which has been most beneficial
  2. Early ambulation, graduated compression stockings, and leg elevation may have a small protective effect. If the patient is confined to bed, bedside physical therapy may be useful.

## REFERENCES

1. Bell WR, Tomasulo PA, Alving BM, et al: Thrombocytopenia occurring during the administration of heparin. Ann Intern Med *85*:155, 1976.
2. Evans BE: Dental treatment of hemophiliacs: Evaluation of dental program (1975–1976) at the Mount Sinai Hospital International Hemophilia Training Center. Mt Sinai J Med *44*:409, 1977.
3. Nunn JF, Freeman J: Problems of oxygenation and oxygen transport during hemorrhage. Anesthesia *19*:206, 1964.
4. Thomas DJ, Marshall J, Russell RWR, et al: Effect of hematocrit on cerebral blood flow in man. Lancet *2*:941, 1977.
5. Wasserman LR, Gilbert, HS: Surgical bleeding in polycythemia vera. Ann NY Acad Sci *115*:112, 1964.
6. International multicenter trial: Prevention of fatal postoperative pulmonary embolism by low doses of heparin. Lancet *2*:45, 1975.
7. Hampson WGJ, Harris FC, Lucas HK, et al: Failure of low-dose heparin to prevent deep vein thrombosis after hip-replacement arthroplasty. Lancet *2*:795, 1974.
8. Sikorski JM, Hampson WG, Staddon GE: The natural history of aetiology of deep vein thrombosis after total hip-replacement. J Bone Joint Surg *63*:171, 1981.
9. Leyvraz PF, Richard J, Bachmann F, et al: Adjusted versus fixed-dose subcutaneous heparin in the prevention of deep-vein thrombosis after total hip-replacement. N Engl J Med *309*:954–958, 1983.
10. Harris WH, Salzman EW, Athanosoulis CA, et al: Aspirin prophylaxis of venous thromboembolism after total hip-replacement. N Engl J Med *297*:1246, 1977.

# 5

# DIABETES MELLITUS

## I. PREOPERATIVE EVALUATION

### A. PURPOSE

1. To assess the degree of metabolic control. The need for closely controlled blood sugar has been well supported, since hyperglycemia may contribute to the development of diabetic ketoacidosis or hyperglycemic hyperosmolar nonketotic coma in the perioperative period. Other risks of hyperglycemia include:
   a. Decreased tensile strength and healing of the wound
   b. Impaired leukocytic phagocytosis
   c. Increased myocardial oxygen demand owing to increased circulating free fatty acids caused by insulin deficiency[1]
2. To identify risk factors and extent of organ damage
3. To identify specific problems, for example:
   a. Extreme sensitivity to insulin
   b. No warning of hypoglycemic symptoms
   c. Allergy to beef insulin
   d. Specific dietary needs
4. To establish therapeutic plan for smooth metabolic control and correction of risk factors when possible

### B. CLINICAL ASSESSMENT

1. History
   The history should be used to help achieve the first three objectives under *Purpose.*
   a. Metabolic control
      Determining the frequency of glucose monitoring and modification of insulin dose by the patient, as well as compliance with diet, will give clues to the level of attention given metabolic control. Polyuria, polydipsia, increased appetite, and other symptoms of hyperglycemia suggest poor control.

b. Identification of risk factors

A list of abnormalities associated with diabetes mellitus is given in Table 5–1. Specific historical information relating to each of these abnormalities should be reviewed. (For a discussion of these abnormalities, see discussion below of risk factors in diabetes.) An assessment of cardiac and vascular diseases is most important, since these are found in a high percentage of diabetics.[2, 3, 4]

c. Specific problems

It is important to identify certain specific problems, such as those listed earlier. These problems are especially common in Type I diabetics. Minor modifications of usual therapeutic regimens will often avoid

**TABLE 5–1. Abnormalities Associated with Increased Surgical Risk in Diabetics**

Vascular disease
  Peripheral
  Cardiac
  Cerebrovascular

Cardiac disease
  Coronary artery disease
  Cardiac autonomic neuropathy

Neuropathy
  Gastroparesis
  Cardiac autonomic neuropathy
  Orthostasis due to autonomic neuropathy

Renal disease
  Reduced renal function (anemia)
  Increase sensitivity to nephrotoxins
  Hyporeninemic hypoaldosteronism
  Nephrotic syndrome

Increased susceptibility to infection
  Lowered cell-mediated immunity
  Reduced phagocytosis

Impaired wound healing

High frequency of obesity

Susceptibility to metabolic disorders
  Fluid shifts
  Acidosis
  Hyperkalemia
  Hypoglycemia

problems in these areas. On the other hand, failing to recognize these problem areas may lead to major complications.

2. Physical examination

The physical examination should be directed toward assessing the abnormalities listed in Table 5–1. Certain neuropathic findings, such as gastroparesis and cardiac autonomic neuropathy, are not commonly found in non-diabetics. Because these findings may be associated with an increased perioperative risk, evidence of their presence must be specifically sought on physical examination.

3. Laboratory assessment

Emphasis should be placed on the evaluation of renal function (creatinine, BUN, electrolytes, urinalysis) and cardiac status (ECG and chest x-ray). Because diabetes is a known risk factor for serious disease in both the kidneys and the heart, even mild abnormalities should be considered carefully. This is especially true for renal disease, as diabetes dramatically increases the susceptibility to nephrotoxins. If serious renal impairment is found, further evaluation of the usual disturbances secondary to renal disease (hematologic and electrolyte abnormalities) is indicated.

Serum glucose determinations should be made fasting and as often as necessary to plan insulin therapy. Bedside fingerstick monitoring is rapidly replacing laboratory glucose monitoring and urine monitoring. The fingerstick method is more accurate than urine monitoring and less expensive and faster than laboratory monitoring. It can be checked easily and often for accurate titration of insulin dosage.

## II. RISK FACTORS IN DIABETES

There is no special formula for estimating risks in diabetes. Rather, the physician must look for the diseases common in diabetics that are known to increase surgical risk. A discussion of some of these abnormalities by organ system follows:

### A. CARDIOVASCULAR DISEASE

1. Diabetics have a high incidence of vascular disease, and the incidence rises with the increasing duration of diabetes.[5] In one study of nearly 400 hospitalized diabetics the incidence went from 20 per cent at 5 years to 60 per cent after 5 to 10 years, to nearly 90 per cent at 20 years.[5]

2. In general, male diabetics have twice the cardiovascular mortality as nondiabetics, whereas for female diabetics the death rate is more than four times as great.[5, 6]

3. Random sampling from a diabetic clinic has shown a 42 per cent incidence of coronary artery disease and a 6.8 per cent incidence of prior myocardial infarction.[7]

4. Patients with cardiac disease have been shown to have four to six times the risk of postoperative infarction as those without.[8, 9]

5. When they do occur, myocardial infarctions in diabetics are more likely to be fatal.[10] In one large series of diabetic surgical patients, 29 per cent of all deaths were from coronary artery disease.[11]

6. Diabetic cardiac denervation apparently accounts for the phenomenon of "painless" myocardial infarction, which is believed to occur in more than 30 per cent of diabetics experiencing an acute event.[12] However, objective evidence documenting a greater prevalence of "silent" myocardial infarction among diabetics has not been reported.[13] The careful historian will usually find that the event is not truly "silent" but may present as atypical pain, nausea, or vomiting, a change in the diabetic equilibrium with elevation in glucose, or onset of congestive heart failure.

Careful evaluation and stabilization of coronary disease is imperative.

## B. NEUROPATHY

1. Cardiac autonomic neuropathy

   Neuropathy affecting the autonomic nervous system can impair cardiac regulation.[14] This has been associated with unexplained postoperative cardiorespiratory arrests[15] and should be suspected in patients with findings of neuropathy involving both the autonomic and peripheral systems (Table 5–2). Tests for this abnormality have been described[16, 17] but are cumbersome and nonspecific. Significant orthostatic blood pressure changes without an appropriate increase in pulse are most suggestive and should be taken as evidence of cardiac involvement.

2. Diabetic gastroparesis

   Gastroparesis is a form of autonomic neuropathy in which stomach emptying is delayed.[18] When this abnormality is present the usual overnight fast may not be sufficient to ensure preoperative stomach emptying, increasing the chances for perioperative vomiting and aspiration. Gastroparesis is detected by placing the fasting

**TABLE 5–2.** Evidence of Neurologic Dysfunction in Diabetics

| Autonomic | Peripheral |
| --- | --- |
| Unexplained resting tachycardia | Decreased vibratory sensation in feet |
| Orthostatic hypotention (15 mm Hg mean) without appropriate increase in pulse | Numbness or pain in extremities |
| Nocturnal diarrhea | Charcot joints |
| Excessive sweating | Foot ulcers |
| Gastroparesis | |

patient in a supine position and auscultating over the stomach while gently rocking the patient from side to side. The presence of a succussion splash indicates inadequate emptying. If gastroparesis is present, the anesthesiologist should be warned and nasogastric suctioning should be considered.

3. Orthostatic hypotension

Orthostatic hypotension is common in diabetics for various reasons. Both autonomic neuropathy and low arterial volume owing to the nephrotic syndrome may be involved. A preoperative evaluation for orthostatic changes in blood pressure should be performed. Extreme care should be exercised when getting a patient out of bed postoperatively if significant orthostatic changes were present preoperatively. A drop in blood pressure may lead to cerebral hypoperfusion and syncope. If the nephrotic syndrome is also present, special care should be taken to avoid inadequate hydration, as this will augment the drop in blood pressure and lead to episodes of syncope.

## C. RENAL DISEASE

1. Reduced renal function and susceptibility to injury

Diabetics have a high incidence of renal disease. A modest reduction in creatinine clearance is not a significant risk factor. However, many reports suggest that diabetics are more sensitive to nephrotoxic renal damage, especially iodinated contrast dyes.[19, 20] The risk of renal damage increases with decreasing renal function and coexisting adverse factors, such as hypertension and exposure to other nephrotoxins.[19, 20, 21] In diabetics with creatinine levels greater than 4.5 mg/dl the risk of dye-induced acute renal failure approaches 100 per cent. Simultaneous nephrotoxic insults should be avoided.

When nephrotoxic agents are to be used, vigorous hydration may reduce the risk of deterioration or renal failure.[21]

2. Nephrotic syndrome

Diabetic renal disease may lead to nephrotic syndrome. Because of the reduced effective arterial volume in this condition, patients require more total body water to maintain adequate arterial perfusion. It is usually appropriate to maintain a trace to 1+ edema in patients with nephrotic syndrome.

3. Hyporeninemic hypoaldosteronism

A small number of diabetics have hyporeninemic hypoaldosteronism. This condition is associated with a mild renal tubular acidosis and moderately elevated potassium. Hyperkalemia can become a problem with (1) coexisting renal insufficiency, (2) acute renal injury, (3) potassium loads, or (4) administration of a potassium-sparing diuretic.

## D. INFECTIONS

Diabetic patients have an increased incidence of infections.[11] More than 13 per cent of the 667 surgical patients reviewed in one series had postoperative infectious complications.[11] In addition to the poor vascular supply to the extremities, an impairment of leukocytic phagocytic function, especially at higher glucose levels, may be partly responsible.[22]

## III. GLUCOSE CONTROL AND METABOLIC CONSIDERATIONS FOR INSULIN-TREATED DIABETICS

Diabetics span a wide range of metabolic lability from the volatile, insulin-sensitive, ketosis-prone Type I patient to the obese, insulin-resistant Type II patient. In their classic forms these may be so different that they deserve individual consideration.

## A. OBJECTIVES OF MANAGEMENT

In treating diabetics through surgery, the goal is to control the metabolic parameters without permitting acidosis or inducing hypoglycemia. Although numerous insulin and glucose regimens have been proposed, there is no ideal protocol. The physician should use the regimen that he or she and the anesthesiologist find most effective in each clinical setting.

## B. TYPE I DIABETICS

1. Insulin sensitivity and metabolic lability

   The variation in metabolic control and response to insulin in ketosis-prone diabetics is so great that even the most experienced physician should seek help from the patient in determining insulin needs. The physician should ask the patient about previous experiences in the hospital. Information about previous hypoglycemic episodes should be specifically sought, as these might indicate extreme sensitivity to regular insulin. Some patients who have been hospitalized may offer valuable suggestions regarding supplementation with regular insulin. It is especially prudent to cooperate with Type I diabetics when they warn against using large doses of regular insulin.

2. Hypoglycemic reactions

   The importance of treating hypoglycemic reactions rapidly cannot be overemphasized. Some patients with volatile glucose regulation and an associated autonomic neuropathy may not have adequate warning of impending hypoglycemic shock. In such patients profound and violent reactions are common and may make glucose administration difficult. For these patients, a 1-mg ampul of glucagon should be kept with their medications for IM injection in an emergency. The glucagon should raise the blood glucose enough to show a clinical response over a 20-minute period. However, attempts to administer IV glucose should not be abandoned.

3. Factors influencing glucose levels

   Multiple factors may influence glucose control in hospitalized diabetics.

   a. Clearly, the pain and physical stress associated with an acute surgical problem will tend to raise glucose levels. Analgesics and rehydration may help when appropriate, but surgical correction is needed. The physician should be alert to the possibility of a dramatic reduction in insulin requirements after a definitive surgical procedure (such as drainage of an abscess) is performed.

   b. Even without physical stress, emotional factors can significantly affect glucose regulation. Insulin requirements may drop dramatically owing to a reduction in anxiety after surgery or at the time of discharge.

   c. A sudden reduction in activity with hospitalization may lead to hyperglycemia despite previous control. This is especially true in young patients in whom activity levels were high before hospitalization.

d. Variable absorption of insulin and calories may affect glucose control. Some patients avoid injections in the arm, as this site is more difficult to reach. The hospital staff frequently use the arm by habit. If usual sites are scarred and fibrotic from heavy use, the change to a relatively unused site sometimes permits a rapid absorption of insulin, leading to hypoglycemia. Additionally, illness leading to hospital admission may also worsen gastroparesis, producing delayed caloric absorption. This leads to the paradoxical appearance of hypoglycemia after meals with hyperglycemia later, when insulin effects are diminished but late absorption begins.

e. The administration of IV glucose may alter laboratory results substantially. Although this source usually represents only a small number of actual calories (1 liter 5% glucose = 200 calories), the direct administration to the blood may have great effects on actual glucose levels. Medications being given in a dextrose solution just before a blood sugar determination may transiently raise levels further, leading to excessive insulin administration.

## C. TYPE II DIABETICS ON INSULIN

Although the principles of evaluation and control are the same for the obese, relatively insulin-resistant diabetic as for Type I patients, metabolic control is usually easier. Aggressive insulin therapy may be undertaken in these patients without the same fear of hypoglycemic reactions. Occasionally, serious illness will produce tremendous insulin resistance in Type II patients requiring large doses of insulin for control. As the underlying condition is corrected, the physician must anticipate a reduction in insulin requirements. It is also noteworthy that caloric restriction frequently increases sensitivity to insulin in these patients. Consequently, patients taking large doses of insulin on admission may require smaller amounts at the time of discharge if caloric restriction occurred during hospitalization.

## D. MANAGEMENT PLANS FOR DIABETICS TREATED WITH INSULIN

1. Special Considerations
   In nearly all cases of routine surgery, management of diabetics is facilitated by having the procedure performed early in the day. This is true for several reasons.

a. Some patients with poor glycogen stores may be sensitive to low levels of insulin. A prolonged fast may deplete stores and lead to a hypoglycemic reaction in the preoperative period.

b. Patients with adequate glycogen stores and gluconeogenic capacity may metabolize all their past doses of insulin, permitting hyperglycemia and acidosis. Administration of insulin to a fasting patient to control this condition is dangerous if caloric intake is not assured.

c. Prolonged waits for surgery in fasting patients lead to dehydration. This can be more serious for some diabetics because of the osmotic diuresis that sometimes occurs, owing to hyperglycemia and glycosuria.

d. The most difficult time for metabolic and fluid control is the immediate postoperative period. Frequent and timely blood glucose determinations as well as careful monitoring for hypoglycemic reactions may not be readily available if the immediate postoperative period stretches into the evening or night hours. If surgery is unavoidably delayed until later in the day, an IV line with glucose should be started in the morning and blood sugars carefully monitored.

2. Insulin and Glucose Schedules

The three basic schedules used for diabetic control during surgery are shown in Table 5–3.

a. No insulin, no glucose

In this schedule no insulin or glucose is given the morning of surgery. Intraoperative fluids contain no dextrose. Blood sugars are checked and regular insulin given as needed until the next morning, when the usual regimen is resumed. This method is usually used for minor procedures, in which the stress is minimal and the patient is expected to eat after surgery.

**TABLE 5–3. Basic Schedules for Diabetic Control During Surgery**

| Preoperative | Postoperative |
|---|---|
| No insulin, no glucose | Foods/insulin as needed |
| Subcutaneous intermediate insulin (50–100% usual dose) plus IV glucose (5–10%) | Subcutaneous regular insulin plus IV glucose |
| Continuous glucose–insulin infusion | Continue glucose–insulin infusion |

(1) Advantages

This regimen is simple and works well for patients who are not labile and whose procedure will not be stressful. It avoids the occasional problem of excessive insulin administration in the fasting preoperative state.

(2) Disadvantages

Disadvantages of this system are seen in patients who become more sensitive to insulin with fasting. Patients with renal disease (which delays insulin catabolism) and those with impaired gluconeogenesis may experience hypoglycemia episodes, especially if surgery is delayed. Others whose disease is labile may become hyperglycemic if insulin activity falls too low.

b. Subcutaneous intermediate insulin and IV glucose

This method is the most common. Usually, one half to two thirds of the usual dose of intermediate insulin is given preoperatively, according to the physician's judgment of the patient's insulin sensitivity and needs. Glucose determinations are made at two- to four-hour intervals. Supplementation with regular insulin is used as needed postoperatively.

(1) Advantages

This method is easy to use and is familiar to most practitioners. It is safe and effective in controlling glucose and acidosis if glucose levels are followed.

(2) Disadvantages

Because this regimen depends on the administration of IV glucose, problems may arise if this access is lost. Such a loss frequently occurs when an IV catheter ruptures a fragile vein during the physical activity of preparing the patient for surgery or for transportation to the operating room. Although the insulin continues to exert its effect, no supplementary glucose is being given. If this condition goes unrecognized, it can lead to a hypoglycemic reaction. Because many diabetics have had repeated venipunctures, venous access may be difficult to establish. Occasionally, floor personnel cannot reestablish access and the physician must interrupt his schedule to ensure continued glucose administration. In patients who go to surgery early to mid-morning, the problem can be avoided by having the insulin administered in the preoperative suite. This way the anesthesiologist can ensure venous access. Because the peak effect of intermediate insulin does not occur for several hours, the anesthesiologist often needs to give supplemental regular insulin during surgery.

c. IV infusion of glucose and insulin

In this technique, insulin and dextrose solution (and sometimes supplemental potassium)[23] are mixed in the IV container and administered simultaneously. Blood glucose is checked frequently over the next four to six hours, and adjustments are made to maintain a stable blood glucose.

(1) Advantages

This technique can be used with all types of diabetics but is most useful in those who are labile or whose surgery is delayed. It prevents wide swings in glucose as well as dehydration. Coadministration of glucose and insulin from the same source prevents the accidental interruption of glucose administration while insulin activity continues (as can happen with injections). If IV access is lost, both insulin and glucose administration stop. The infusion prevents problems with variable insulin absorption and provides smoother metabolic control than is possible with the peaks and troughs of injected insulin.

(2) Disadvantages

This technique has several drawbacks. Although experimental evidence shows that superior metabolic control is possible, many physicians are unfamiliar with this method. Adjusting concentration and flow rates is not always a simple matter, and overall satisfactory results may not be achieved by inexperienced clinicians. If the patient is poorly controlled before surgery, four or five preoperative changes in insulin administration rate may be necessary to arrive at a steady state. This can mean changing the IV solution frequently merely to add or subtract several units of insulin. The problem can be overcome by using an insulin pump, but this increases the chance for improper use or breakdown of equipment. When frequent changes are anticipated, a reasonable compromise can be achieved by using two IV bottles of dextrose solution—one with double the usual insulin concentration and one without insulin. These can be connected into a main line so that the rate of infusion of either solution can be adjusted to optimize metabolic control. Although some insulin may adhere to the IV apparatus,[24] this rarely exceeds 35 per cent to 40 per cent of the insulin activity.[25] This effect can be easily overcome by increasing the infusion rate or increasing insulin concentration.

3. Comparison of management plans for diabetics on insulin
  a. Experimental data on insulin techniques for surgery
      An experimental comparison of metabolic control of the three management plans has been done to determine effectiveness of glucose control and keto acid production in surgical patients.[23] Both the no-insulin and the intermediate-insulin plans permit significant elevations in serum levels of glucose and keto acids (although keto acids are higher in the no-insulin approach). The glucose–insulin infusion provides better control of both these parameters than do the other techniques. The authors have concluded that the glucose–insulin infusion provides the best metabolic control. With the infusion method, however, transient loss of control has been noted in some patients in the immediate postoperative period. Additionally, other authors using this technique have noted rapid falls in blood sugar, suggesting that this technique may not be appropriate when less careful observation is anticipated.

      There are no data to show that any particular degree of control of glucose or ketone bodies alters the outcome of surgery. Although one of the preceding techniques may be more appropriate for some situations, the physician should adopt the techniques he or she and the anesthesiologist are most comfortable with. Despite the method used, it is still necessary to monitor serum glucose frequently and to adjust therapy appropriately.[26]

## E. SPECIFIC RECOMMENDATIONS FOR THE MANAGEMENT OF INSULIN-TREATED DIABETICS

1. Major surgery
  a. Stable Type I diabetics
      Stable Type I diabetics can be treated preoperatively with one half to two thirds of the usual intermediate dose of insulin and an IV infusion of 5% dextrose

begun. Serum glucose should be monitored frequently (every four to six hours), giving either regular insulin or combinations of regular and intermediate-acting insulin as needed. Insulin coverage based on blood sugars should be continued until the patient is eating and his or her normal schedule can be resumed.

As discussed earlier, coverage (which may be on a sliding scale) should be based on blood sugars. Coverage based on urine sugars (inaccurate because of wide variations in renal threshhold) has become passé with the ready availability of fingerstick monitoring.

b. Unstable Type I diabetics

Some unstable Type I diabetics are difficult to control with subcutaneous injections. Such patients are most conveniently treated by glucose–insulin infusion. We recommend the use of 10 units of regular insulin in 1000 ml of 5% dextrose to run at a rate of 100 ml/h. This is only a starting point and should be initiated 6 to 12 hours before surgery to provide time for sufficient glucose determinations to establish a satisfactory infusion rate. Woodruff and associates[1] have described a technique that can achieve and maintain strict blood glucose control in patients who have severe hyperglycemia the morning of surgery. Their algorithm consists of continuous low-dose glucose infusion (100 mg/kg/h) and variable insulin infusion rates (as noted in Table 5–4) based on glucose level (checked every 15 minutes using glucose analyzers).

Because of the short half-life of regular insulin, this system should be continued until it is appropriate to begin using subcutaneous intermediate insulin. We prefer to stop the infusions only in the mornings when intermediate insulin is begun (or patient's normal schedule is resumed).

**TABLE 5–4. Insulin Infusion Rates for Rapid Correction of Hyperglycemia**

| Serum Glucose (mg/dl) | Continuous Insulin Infusion Rates (units/hr)* |
|---|---|
| <80 | 0 |
| 80–200 | 1 |
| >200 | 20 |

*50 units regular insulin in 250 ml of normal saline

c. Type II diabetics on insulin

For Type II diabetics, especially if obese, give one half to two thirds of the usual dose of intermediate insulin. For patients scheduled in the morning, it is our approach to give the intermediate-acting insulin "on-call" to the operating room or actually in the preoperative room to avoid problems with venous access. The intermediate insulin primarily smoothes the postoperative course and should not be expected to be sufficient for complete intraoperative or postoperative control. Regular insulin supplementation is given, according to blood sugar determinations, every four to six hours in an attempt to keep glucose levels between 140 to 200 mg/100 ml. For patients requiring less than 20 units of insulin in their usual regimen, we are more conservative with the initial insulin dose. Alternatively, a glucose–insulin infusion may be used, particularly if blood sugars are high on the morning of surgery. However, we rarely find it necessary to use this alternative with such patients.

2. Minor surgery

Many options are available for the insulin-dependent patient undergoing minor surgery, based on blood sugar and duration of surgery.

In long procedures IV glucose should be administered and one-half to two-thirds of the normal intermediate-acting insulin given. Insulin needs for the remainder of the day may be satisfied by giving the remainder of the patient's intermediate-acting insulin dose postoperatively or by covering with regular insulin. This decision can be made based on blood sugars and the patient's ability to eat.

## IV. GLUCOSE AND METABOLIC CONSIDERATIONS FOR TYPE II DIABETICS ON ORAL HYPOGLYCEMIC AGENTS

### A. OBJECTIVES OF MANAGEMENT

The goals of therapy in diabetics taking oral agents are identical to those of insulin-dependent diabetics except that acidosis is not a problem. The complicating feature with these patients is that their baseline response to insulin, which will be required for major surgery, is unknown. Until the baseline response can be established, this factor may increase the risk of hyperglycemia from undertreatment or the risk of hypoglycemia from aggressive treatment.

B. **SPECIFIC RECOMMENDATIONS FOR THE MANAGEMENT OF TYPE II DIABETICS ON ORAL HYPOGLYCEMIC AGENTS**

1. Major surgery
   a. When possible, an insulin regimen should be initiated several days before surgery in an effort to determine insulin requirements and stabilize blood glucose levels. One half to two thirds of the intermediate-acting insulin can then be given on call to the operating room and the patient can be managed with regular insulin based on blood sugar determinations every six hours postoperatively.
   b. When insulin therapy cannot be initiated before surgery, regular insulin therapy is begun during surgery with frequent glucose monitoring.
   c. A glucose–insulin infusion may be used alternatively, particularly if blood sugars are high on the morning of surgery.
   d. Oral hypoglycemics may be restarted when normal diet is resumed.
   e. Because of the theoretical concern over the induction of insulin antibodies in patients not taking insulin,[27] we use human insulin.
2. Minor surgery
   a. For diabetics on oral hypoglycemic agents undergoing minor surgery, we withhold the medication on the day of surgery. If the surgery is early in the morning and the patient is eating postoperatively, the oral agent is resumed. If surgery is delayed or the patient is expected to be NPO for many hours, an IV line with dextrose is started, blood glucose is monitored, and regular insulin (human) is given if needed.

## V. DIABETIC KETOACIDOSIS

### A. PRIMARY OBJECTIVES OF TREATMENT

The treatment of diabetic ketoacidosis has been discussed extensively[28, 29] and will not be reviewed here. The primary objectives of treatment of the patient with ketoacidosis are more important preoperatively. These are:

1. To identify the precipitating cause and correct it if possible.

2. To correct the acidosis
3. To correct the hypovolemia
4. To correct the hyperglycemia
5. To monitor carefully and correct the electrolyte abnormalities known to occur with diabetic ketoacidosis and its therapy (e.g., hypokalemia and hypophosphatemia)
6. To avoid excessive therapy (hypoglycemia)
7. To support failed systems (cardiac, respiratory, or renal failure)

## B. IMPORTANT CORRECTABLE RISK FACTORS IN KETOACIDOSIS

Although it is never appropriate to operate electively on a patient in acidosis, this condition may be impossible to correct in cases in which the precipitating event requires surgical correction. When this is true, delay may be counterproductive. However, a transient partial correction of certain factors known to adversely affect surgical risk may be accomplished.

1. Acidosis

Acidosis has the effect of causing arterial dilatation, of blunting the response of the heart and blood vessels to catecholamines, and of depressing neural activity throughout the body.[30, 31] These effects increase in importance as the pH becomes depressed below 7.2 and may become profound as the pH approaches 7.0.[30] The acidosis of diabetic ketoacidosis nearly always responds well to insulin and fluids. Bicarbonate administration is indicated only for (1) coma, shock, hypotension accompanying a pH of 7.2 or less and for (2) a pH of less than 7.1. Sodium bicarbonate is given as two ampuls (total of 88 mEq) in 1 liter of 0.45% sodium chloride, given over the first hour and repeated until the pH reaches 7.2 and the patient no longer is in shock.

2. Hypovolemia

The patient in diabetic ketoacidosis has multiple causes for reduced intravascular volume. These include an osmotic diuresis, lack of oral intake, increased insensible loss owing to hyperventilation, and fluid sequestration at the site of the surgical disease. If hypovolemia is combined with the cardiac depressant and hypotensive effects of anesthesia, as well as with the reduced ability of the cardiovascular system to compensate during acidosis, as mentioned earlier, profound tissue hypoperfusion may result. Insertion of a central line for pressure monitoring and the rapid repletion of intravascular volume should be accomplished in any patient who must undergo emergency surgery.

3. Hyperkalemia

High potassium values can promote heart block and adversely affect the propagation of the cardiac action potential.[32] Although the seriousness of this problem varies with individual cases, a rapidly rising potassium greater than 7.5 mEq/L can be extremely dangerous.[32, 33] Therapy with alkali, insulin, fluids, and, if ECG abnormalities are present, 10 ml of 10% calcium gluconate IV can be undertaken for rapid but transient improvement of the effects of hyperkalemia on the heart.

## REFERENCES

1. Woodruff RE, Lewis S, McLeskey CH et al.: Avoidance of surgical hyperglycemia in diabetic patients. JAMA 244:166, 1980.
2. Steinke J, Soeldner JS: Diabetes mellitus, in Thorn et al (eds): Harrison's Textbook of Medicine. New York, McGraw-Hill, 1975, p 564.
3. Rabinowitz D, Lockwood D, Prut T, et al: Diabetes mellitus, in Harvey et al (eds): The Principles and Practice of Medicine. East Norwalk, Appleton-Century-Crofts, 1972, p 879.
4. Porte D, Halter J: The endocrine pancreas and diabetes mellitus, in Williams RH (ed): Textbook of Endocrinology, 6th ed. Philadelphia, WB Saunders, 1981.
5. Bryfogle JW, Bradley RF: The vascular complications of diabetes mellitus. A clinical study. Diabetes 6:159, 1957.
6. Garcia MJ, McNamara PM, Gordon T, et al: Morbidity and mortality in diabetics in the Framingham population study. 16-year follow-up study. Diabetes 23:105, 1974.
7. Liebow IM, Hellerstein HK, Miller M: Arteriosclerotic heart disease in diabetes mellitus. A clinical study of 383 patients. Am J Med 18:438, 1955.
8. Knapp RB, Tompkins MJ, Artusio JF: The cerebrovascular accident and coronary occlusion in anesthesia. JAMA 182:106, 1962.
9. Tarhan S, Moffitt EA, Taylor WF et al: Myocardial infarction after general anesthesia. JAMA 220:1451, 1972.
10. Solar NG, Pentecost BL, Bennett MA, et al: Coronary care for myocardial infarction in diabetics. Lancet 1:475, 1974.
11. Galloway JA, Schuman CR: Diabetes in surgery. A study of 667 cases. Am J Med 34:177, 1963.
12. Gregerman RI: Metabolic and endocrine problems in Barker LR, Burton JR, Zieve PD (eds): Principles of Ambulatory Medicine. Baltimore, Williams & Wilkins, 1982, p 700.
13. Felig P, et al (eds): Endocrinology and Metabolism. New York: McGraw-Hill, 1981, p 826.
14. Page MM, Watkins PJ: The heart in diabetes: Autonomic neuropathy in cardiomyopathy. Clin Endocrinol Metab 6:337, 1977.

15. Page MM, Watkins PJ: Cardiorespiratory arrest and diabetic autonomic neuropathy. Lancet *1*:14, 1978.
16. Fraser DM, Campbell IW, Ewing DJ, et al: Peripheral and autonomic nerve function in newly diagnosed diabetes mellitus. Diabetes *36*:456, 1977.
17. Ewing DJ, Campbell IW, Murray A, et al: Immediate heart-rate response to standing; simple test for autonomic neuropathy in diabetics. Br Med J *1*:145, 1978.
18. Zitomer BR, Gramm HF, Kozak GP: Gastric neuropathy in diabetes mellitus; Clinical and radiographic observations. Metabolism *17*:199, 1968.
19. VanZee BE, Hay WE, Tolley TE, et al: Renal injury associated with intravenous pyelography in nondiabetic and diabetic patients. Ann Intern Med *89*:51, 1978.
20. Harkonen S, Kjellstrand CM: Exacerbation of diabetic renal failure following intravenous pyelography. Am J Med *63*:939, 1977.
21. Rose BD: Acute renal failure, in Pathophysiology of Renal Disease. New York, McGraw-Hill, 1981, pp 55.
22. Bagdade JD, Nielson KL, Gulger RJ: Reversible abnormalities in phagocytic function in poorly controlled diabetic patients. Am J Med Sci *263*:431, 1972.
23. Alberti KGMM, Thomas DJV: The management of diabetes during surgery. Br J Anaesth *51*:693, 1979.
24. Weisenfeld S, Podolsky S, Goldsmith L, et al: Absorption of insulin to infusion bottles and tubing. Diabetes *17*:766, 1968.
25. Hirsch JI, Fratkin MJ, Wood JH, et al: Clinical significance of insulin absorption by polyvinyl chloride infusion systems. Am J Hosp Pharm *34*:583, 1977.
26. Walts LF, Miller J, Davidson MD, et al: Perioperative management of diabetes mellitus. Anesthesiology *55*:104, 1981.
27. Asplin CM, Hartog M, Goldia DJ: Change of insulin dosage, circulating free and bound insulin, and insulin antibodies on transferring diabetics from conventional to highly purified porcine insulin. Diabetologia *14*:99, 1978.
28. Bradley RF: Treatment of diabetic ketoacidosis in coma. Med Clin North Am *49*:961, 1965.
29. Sacks HS, Shahshahani M, Kitabchi AE, et al: Similar responsiveness of diabetic ketoacidosis to low-dose insulin by intramuscular injection and albumin-free infusion. Ann Intern Med *90*:36, 1979.
30. Thrower WD, Darby TD, Aldinger EE: Acid-based arrangements in myocardial contractility. Arch Surg *82*:76, 1961.
31. Guyton AC: Affects of acidosis and alkalosis on the body, in Textbook of Medical Physiology. Philadelphia, WB Saunders, 1969, p 524.
32. Chung, EK: Digitalis and electrolyte imbalances, in Electrocardiography: Practical Applications with Vectorial Principles. Hagerstown, Harper & Row, 1974, p 496.
33. Feldman MS, Helfant RH: Disturbances of electrolyte balance, in Helfant RH (ed): Bellet's Essentials of Cardiac Arrhythmias. Philadelphia, WB Saunders, 1980, p 276.

# 6

# THYROID DISEASE

## I. HYPERTHYROIDISM

### A. PREOPERATIVE EVALUATION

1. Purpose
   a. To determine the state of thyroid function
   b. To identify end-organ effects due to thyroid dysfunction. These may be viewed in two distinct categories: those resulting from catecholamine effects and those resulting from protein turnover effects (see Table 6–1). The catecholamine effects represent the most acute and immediate risks to the surgical patient. These can be controlled in a matter of hours through the use of beta blocking agents. The protein turnover effects particularly contribute to risks of poor healing and delayed recovery time and may take months to correct once thyroid function is normalized.
   c. To bring the patient to surgery in the euthyroid state for elective surgery, or symptomatically controlled as well as possible for emergency surgery
2. Clinical assessment
   a. History and physical examination
      (1) The history and physical examination are aimed at identifying the signs and symptoms listed in Table 6–1.
      (2) The frequency of these signs and symptoms are reviewed in Table 6–2. Unfortunately, the most common symptoms (nervousness, sweating, palpitations, fatigue, tachycardia) are not specific and often may occur in patients who are anxious. Probably the most difficult task facing the physician is the frequent need to accurately, but rapidly, exclude hyperthyroidism in the anxious preoperative patient.

**TABLE 6–1. Effects of Hyperthyroidism**

| Excess Beta Stimulation | Excessive Catabolism |
|---|---|
| Insomnia | Weight loss |
| Anxiety | Myopathy (proximal) |
| Tremor | Increased metabolic rate |
| Tachycardia | Increased appetite |
| Palpitations | Cardiomyopathy |
| Increased cardiac output | Osteoporosis |
| Increased cardiac contractility | Hypercalciuria |
| Increased sweating | Hypercalcemia |
| Wide pulse pressure | |
| Lid lag | |
| Abnormal glucose tolerance test | |

**TABLE 6–2. Incidence of Signs and Symptoms of Hyperthyroidism**

| Symptoms | Percentage of Patients |
|---|---|
| Nervousness | 99 |
| Hyperhidrosis | 91 |
| Hypersensitivity to heat | 89 |
| Palpitations | 89 |
| Fatigue | 88 |
| Weight loss | 85 |
| Tachycardia | 82 |
| Dyspnea | 75 |
| Weakness | 70 |
| Hyperorexia | 65 |
| Eye complaints | 54 |
| Leg swelling | 35 |
| Diarrhea | 23 |
| **Signs** | |
| Tachycardia | 100 |
| Goiter | 100 |
| Skin changes | 97 |
| Tremor | 97 |
| Bruit over thyroid | 77 |
| Eye signs | 71 |
| Thyroid heart | 15 |
| Auricular fibrillation | 10 |
| Splenomegaly | 10 |
| Gynecomastia | 10 |
| Liver palms | 8 |

From Williams RH: Thiouracil treatment of thyrotoxicosis, in The results of prolonged treatment. J Clin Endocrinol 6:1, 1946.

Because thyroid function tests are often unavailable before surgery, the patient must be observed for certain clues to help the physician decide when delay is appropriate. The presence of long-term symptoms, such as increased appetite, weight loss, and hypersensitivity to heat, should raise the index of suspicion. In addition, such physical findings as goiter, tremor, thyroid bruits, and eye signs make the diagnosis more likely. A persistence of the tachycardia after sedation or while the patient is asleep is another indication that symptoms are not caused by anxiety alone. When several of these signs are present and tachycardia persists during sleep, surgery should be delayed until thyroid function tests are obtained.

One must remember, however, that even when hyperthyroidism is not present, other etiologies for the signs and symptoms of excess adrenergic stimulation should be considered. Alcohol or drug withdrawal, excessive beta stimulator therapy, infection, hypoglycemia, and even a pheochromocytoma could give rise to these symptoms and adversely affect surgical outcome. One should make every effort to consider other conditions consistent with these findings. In cases in which other serious underlying medical problems, such as pulmonary or cardiac disease, already exist, it becomes imperative to diagnose and control even mild hyperthyroidism preoperatively.

b. Laboratory assessment

The most helpful tests are serum thyroxine ($T_4$), $T_3$ resin uptake ($T_3RU$), and serum triiodothyronine measured by radioimmunoassay ($T_3RIA$). TSH (thyroid-stimulating hormone) is not helpful in making the diagnosis of hyperthyroidism. Normal values are listed in Table 6–3.

(1) Serum $T_4$

The serum $T_4$, which is the most commonly used screening test, will be elevated in about 90 per cent of hyperthyroid patients.[1] It is a measure of the total protein-bound and unbound thyroxine. Although the majority of $T_4$ is bound to thyroxine-binding globulin (TBG), it is the tiny unbound fraction (about 0.025 per cent) that is physiologically active. This unbound $T_4$ fraction is main-

TABLE 6–3. Approximate Normal Values for Thyroid Function
Tests

| $T_4$ | $T_3$ RU | $T_3$ RIA | TSH |
|---|---|---|---|
| 4.5–12.5 | 35–45% | 65–190 | <10 |

tained nearly constant in euthyroid individuals.
Under certain circumstances an increase in the
production of TBG can occur. In order to maintain
equilibrium when this occurs, more $T_4$ will be
produced and bound to TBG, resulting in an
increase in the measured $T_4$. However, the amount
of physiologically active $T_4$ remains constant.

(2) $T_3$ resin uptake

To avoid erroneous diagnoses when the $T_4$ is
elevated, the amount of TBG should be estimated
by the $T_3$RU. In this test the value obtained is
essentially the reciprocal estimate of the unoccu-
pied binding sites on TBG. When the value is
high, most TBG binding sites are occupied by $T_4$.
When it is low, many sites are available. When
combined with a high $T_4$ value, a low $T_3$RU
suggests that many TBG binding sites are available
despite the high $T_4$. Therefore, the elevated $T_4$ is
most likely related to an overproduction of TBG.
When a high $T_3$RU accompanies a high $T_4$, most
binding sites are saturated and therefore $T_4$ is
probably being overproduced.

(3) Free thyroxine index

Because the $T_4$ and TBG vary inversely in
euthyroid patients, the product of the $T_4$ and the
decimal value of $T_3$RU (known as the $T_7$, or free
thyroxine index) has been found to fall in fairly
constant range in most euthyroid patients. By
using these two tests to determine the amount of
$T_4$ and TBG, most cases of hyperthyroidism can
be differentiated from altered normal states. Because the $T_4$ is elevated in more than 90 per cent
of hyperthyroid patients, it can be used alone as
a screening test when time is not a factor. The
$T_3$RU may then be done if the $T_4$ is found to be
elevated.

(4) Serum $T_3$ ($T_3$ by radioimmunoassay)

Much less commonly, serum $T_4$ levels will be
normal in hyperthyroid individuals who have an

elevated serum $T_3$. This "$T_3$ toxicosis" is seen more often in older patients, in patients who have been treated for hyperthyroidism, and in the early phases of thyrotoxicosis. In some cases it may result from thyrotoxicosis that has been discovered early, before the $T_4$ has risen above normal. When clinical suspicion is high but the $T_7$ is only in the upper normal range, the $T_3RIA$ should be checked. The $T_3RIA$ is the most sensitive test for thyrotoxicosis, but levels can be low in thyrotoxic patients who are acutely ill or malnourished.[2] The common factors affecting thyroid function studies are summarized in Table 6–4.

## B. SURGICAL RISK FACTORS

1. Cardiac arrhythmias

    Cardiac arrhythmias are common with hyperthyroidism. Virtually 100 per cent of patients have tachycardia and 10 per cent have atrial fibrillation before therapy.[3] These patients are relatively resistant to digoxin and other antiarrhythmic medication until returned to the euthyroid state.[4, 5] Beta blockers are often effective in helping control arrhythmias.

2. Malnutrition

    Malnutrition and a state of negative nitrogen balance occur frequently owing to the excessive catabolism. Increased degradation of protein, vitamins, and anabolic hormones, such as insulin, are contributory. As in any patient, this reduces the rate of wound healing and may increase susceptibility to infection.

**TABLE 6–4. Factors Affecting Common Thyroid Function Tests**

| Factor | $T_4$ | $T_3$ RIA | $T_3$ RU | TSH |
|---|---|---|---|---|
| Normal | N | N | N | N |
| Hyperthyroid | ↑ | ↑ | ↑ | ↑ ↓ |
| Hypothyroid | | | | |
|   Primary (common) | ↓ | ↓ | ↓ | ↑ |
|   Secondary (rare) | ↓ | ↓ | ↓ | ↓ |
| Pregnancy, estrogens ( ↑ TBG) | ↑ | ↑ or N | ↓ | N |
|   androgens, starvation ( ↓ TBG) | ↓ | N | ↑ | N |
| Phenytoin, aspirin (drug binding to TBG) | ↓ | N or ↓ | ↑ | N |

3. Myopathy

A myopathy associated with hyperthyroidism can impair pulmonary function and increase pulmonary complications in postoperative patients. Ventilator weaning may be impaired. Muscle weakness may also impair postoperative mobilization and increase the complications associated with bed rest, such as atelectasis and pneumonia.

4. Thyroid storm (see discussion later in this chapter)

## C. MANAGEMENT OF THE HYPERTHYROID PATIENT UNDERGOING NONTHYROID SURGERY

1. Elective surgery

   a. A euthyroid state should always be achieved before elective surgery.

   b. Any evidence of poor nutritional status, myopathy, or cardiac disease must be reversed before surgery. Such reversal may take weeks to months.

   c. Medical management (see Tables 6–5 and 6–6 for dosages and synopsis of therapeutic agents)

      (1) Propylthiouracil or methimazole are used in the indicated dosages to return the patient to euthyroidism. Once euthyroid, there is no chance of thyroid storm and the patient is free of the catabolic effects that cannot be completely controlled by beta blockade. However, problems include occasional allergic reactions to the drugs as well as rare (less than 0.2 per cent) and usually reversible agranulocytosis. Additionally, propylthiouracil crosses the placenta, enabling it to cause goiter and toxic reactions in the fetus. Finally, the period of preparation using these drugs is 4 to 12 weeks. In severe cases, as well as some cases of pregnancy, full control may not be achieved.[6]

      Temporary discontinuation of antithyroid drugs postoperatively generally presents no problem, but if oral intake is interrupted for longer than three days, the medication should be crushed and instilled through a nasogastric tube if the bowel is functioning. The patient should be covered with beta blockers during this time.

      (2) Beta blocking agents, such as propranolol, are commonly used as adjunctive therapy to control adrenergic hyperactivity. Such agents generally should not be used alone, since thyroid storm has been reported.[7, 8] However, in the patient who

**TABLE 6–5. Dosage Regimens for Surgery in the Hyperthyroid Patient**

| | |
|---|---|
| Preop: | Propylthiouracil: 100–150 mg PO q8h or methimazole 5–15 mg q8h.<br>Propranolol: 10–80 mg PO q.i.d. (to control pulse < 80 beats/min)<br>SSKI: 1–2 drops (50–100 mg) PO q8h. |
| Postop: | Resume when patient is able to take oral medication, or crush and give by nasogastric tube for unconscious patient. Withholding drug for several days usually will not cause exacerbation. |

**Emergency**

| | |
|---|---|
| Preop: | Propylthiouracil: 600–1000 mg initial dose, followed by 150–200 mg PO or by nasogastric tube q4–6h.<br>Propranolol: 20–80 mg PO q4–6h, or 1–5 mg IV q4–6h as needed to control adrenergic stimulation before and during surgery SSKI: 2–5 drops PO, q8h or sodium iodide 1 gm IV q8h to block thyroid hormone release. Should be started two hours after propylthiouracil.<br>Dexamethasone: 2 mg IV q6h for four doses, to decrease hormonal release and block peripheral $T_4$ to $T_3$ conversion. |
| Postop: | Resume propylthiouracil PO or by nasogastric tube in 100–200-mg dose q6–8h as soon as possible postop, with eventual reduction to maintenance dose.<br>Continue IV propranolol 1–5 mg IV q6h until PO medication can be resumed.<br>Continue sodium iodide 1 gm IV q8h until SSKI can be given 1–2 drops PO q8h. |

cannot tolerate propylthiouracil or methimazole, surgery usually can be safely performed using propranolol alone or with iodine preparation.[6, 8, 9] Beta blockage has the advantage of rapid symptomatic relief and control of excess adrenergic stimulation. Coswell and co-workers[6] were able to control symptoms and signs in four pregnant patients with beta blockage, when they were unable to do so completely with antithyroid agents. However, prolonged administration of propranolol to pregnant women may be associated with fetal abnormalities.[10, 11] Contraindications include asthma, heart failure, and possibly, brittle diabetes.

(3) SSKI (supersaturated potassum iodide) may also be used adjunctively.

**TABLE 6–6. Drugs Used in the Treatment of Hyperthyroidism**

| Agent | Action | Benefits | Problems |
|---|---|---|---|
| Propylthiouracil | ↓ Synthesis<br>↓ Peripheral conversion $T_4$ to $T_3$ | ↓ $T_4$ ↓ $T_3$<br>↓ Symptoms<br>↓ Protein turnover<br>Single agent | Rash<br>Agranulocytosis (reversible)<br>Crosses placenta<br>No ↓ vascularity<br>Oral only |
| Methimazole | ↓ Synthesis only | As above, but no peripheral effect | |
| Iodine SSKI<br>Sodium iodide | ↓ Hormone release (block organification) | ↓ Vascularity<br>Rapid effect | Possible escape<br>Gland immune to $I^{131}$ and antithyroid agent for several weeks<br>Not single agent |
| Beta blockers | Beta blockade | Rapid effect<br>Single agent | Contraindicated in asthma and CHF<br>Impairs gluconeogenesis<br>Incomplete control of protein turnover<br>Thyroid storm reported but rare |
| Steroids | ↓ Peripheral conversion and release | Provides steroid cover for adrenal deficiency<br>↓ Peripheral conversion | Potential steroid problems<br>↑ BP ↑ Glucose<br>Short-term use avoids chronic complications |

2. Emergency surgery in uncontrolled hyperthyroidism
   a. Goals are to reduce thyroid hormone levels and adrenergic hyperactivity rapidly. These factors may precipitate thyroid storm.
   b. Propylthiouracil is preferred over methimazole in this situation because of its ability to inhibit conversion of $T_4$ to $T_3$ in addition to inhibiting hormone synthesis.
   c. The full dosage regimen in Table 6–5 for emergency surgery should be instituted. Adrenergic symptoms will largely be controlled and $T_3$ levels halved in 24 to 48 hours. If surgery is indicated within a few hours, IV propranolol should be given with close cardiac monitoring.

3. Thyroid storm
   a. The gravest complication facing the hyperthyroid patient is the development of thyroid storm. Although this entity has become uncommon since the development of adequate methods of prevention, it remains important because of the 20 per cent to 40 per cent mortality associated with its occurrence.[5] When thyroid storm is precipitated by the stress of major surgery, it will most likely occur in the patient with unrecognized or inadequately treated hyperthyroidism who comes unexpectedly to the operating room. However, some cases have been reported after even minor surgical procedures in patients whose disease was felt to be sufficiently mild that no therapy was required. As mentioned earlier, some cases have also been reported in which thyroid storm developed in patients who were felt to be adequately controlled on beta blockers.[7]

   Nearly all cases occur immediately postoperatively. Clinically, thyroid storm is recognized by sudden rise in temperature (to more than 100° F) with a disproportionately increased heart rate. The primary systems involved are the cardiovascular and central nervous systems. Arrhythmias are common, but the high-output type of congestive heart failure is seen primarily in patients with underlying heart disease. Central nervous system manifestations include agitation, psychosis, stupor, and coma. When thyroid storm occurs after surgery, it almost always is seen within several hours. Fever and tachycardia, which begin more than 24 hours after surgery, most likely result from another cause.[12]

   Stresses other than surgery that may precipitate thyroid storm include infection, septicemia, trauma, dehydration, diabetic ketoacidosis, severe fright, rapid iodine withdrawal, and radioiodine contrast studies.

b. Therapy for thyroid storm is the same as that described for emergency surgery of the thyrotoxic patient, in Table 6–5. However, additional supportive care is critical. Careful fluid and electrolyte replacement through IV lines is indicated owing to fluid loss from fever and diaphoresis. Increased caloric demands require glucose and vitamin therapy. Oxygen should be provided to meet increased metabolic demand; cooling blankets may be required for hyperthermia. High-output congestive heart failure may occur and may be exacerbated by beta blockers. In this situation, hemo-dynamic monitoring is essential.

## D. SPECIAL CONSIDERATIONS IN THE PATIENT UNDER-GOING THYROIDECTOMY

1. Medical therapy is essentially the same as for any patient with hyperthyroidism undergoing surgery, as outlined earlier. Because this type of surgery is always elective, an euthyroid state should be attained using propylthiouracil or methimazole several weeks before surgery. Gland vascularity and friability should be reduced by using SSKI, 1 to 2 drops t.i.d. for one to two weeks before surgery, in conjunction with propranolol 10 to 80 mg q.i.d. Thyroidectomy can be performed using these two modalities alone if propylthiouracil or methimazole is not tolerated, although risk of thyroid storm is increased.[13]

2. Certain complications of thyroid surgery should be expected in a percentage of cases. The incidence of some of the more common complications is shown in Table 6–7. Most frequently, one could expect to see hypoparathyroidism, vocal cord paralysis, and bleeding into the operative site.[4, 14] Complications often are related to the

**TABLE 6–7. Incidence of Complications in Surgery for Hyperthyroidism***

| Complication | Percentage |
|---|---|
| Mortality | 0.0–3.1 |
| Recurrent hyperthyroidism | 0.6–17.9 |
| Vocal cord paralysis | 0.0–4.4 |
| Permanent hypoparathyroidism | 0.0–3.6 |
| Permanent hypothyroidism | 4.0–29.7 |

From Hershman JM: The treatment of hyperthyroidism. Ann Intern Med *64*:1306, 1966.
*As reported from eight clinics.

experience of the surgeon, and in sending any patient for thyroid surgery, this should be strongly considered.

a. Bleeding

Excessive bleeding at the operative site requires immediate evacuation and control of the bleeding vessel, as pressure on the trachea can lead to asphyxiation.

b. Vocal cord paralysis

Vocal cord paralysis, which may occur in up to 4.4 per cent of cases, may leave the patient permanently hoarse.

c. Hypoparathyroidism

This condition may be either transient or permanent, depending on the amount of parathyroid tissue removed and damage to the blood supply of the glands that remain. Hypocalcemia will usually appear within one to seven days after the operation. Symptoms may include depression, paresthesias, and heightened neuromuscular activity, such as Chvostek's and Trousseau's signs. Serum calcium should be checked daily. The finding of an extremely low serum calcium with clinical evidence of neuromuscular excitability is an indication for calcium replacement. Treatment should consist of 10 to 20 ml of 10% calcium gluconate over a 10-minute period. This may be repeated every four to eight hours as needed to control symptoms. In milder cases oral calcium chloride, 1 gm three times daily, can be used. Hypoparathyroidism may improve within a few weeks after surgery.

## II. HYPOTHYROIDISM

### A. PREOPERATIVE EVALUATION

1. Purpose
   a. To determine the state of thyroid function
   b. To identify end-organ effects due to thyroid dysfunction. This may involve every organ system, as outlined in Table 6–8. Many effects may be thought to be related to surgery if not recognized previously.
   c. To bring the patient to surgery in the euthyroid state, with correction of end-organ and metabolic abnormalities

2. Clinical assessment
   a. History and physical examination
      (1) In most cases the onset of symptoms is gradual, and they are not presented as complaints. (The

**TABLE 6–8. Effects of Hypothyroidism**

| Heart | Lungs | Vascular |
|---|---|---|
| Pericardial effusion | Pleural effusions | Hypotension |
| Bradycardia | Myxedematous | ↑ Peripheral |
| ↓ Cardiac output | infiltration of | vascular |
| ↓ Stroke volume | respiratory | resistance |
| ↑ Incidence of | muscles | ↓ Blood volume |
| ischemic heart | Depression of | ↑ Atherosclerosis |
| disease | respiratory | with ↑ BP |
| Administration of | center | |
| thyroxine and | Alveolar hypo- | |
| vasopressors lead to | ventilation | |
| ventricular | ↓ Responsiveness | |
| fibrillation | of respiratory | |
| Blood loss poorly | center to | |
| tolerated | hypoxia and | |
| ↑ CPK, LDH, SGOT | hypoventilation | |

| Renal | CNS | Hematologic |
|---|---|---|
| ↓ Renal blood flow | ↓ Blood flow but | ↓ Platelet |
| ↓ GFR | normal oxygen | adhesiveness |
| ↓ Excretion water | consumption | Pernicious anemia |
| load | ↓ Respiratory | |
| Disordered vasopressin | center | |
| secretion | responsiveness to | |
| Hyponatremia | ↓ $O_2$ and ↑ | |
| | $CO_2$ | |
| | ↑ Sensitivity to | |
| | sedation | |
| | ↑ Cerebral | |
| | atherosclerosis | |
| | Seizures (in | |
| | myxedema | |
| | coma) | |

| Other Endocrine | Other |
|---|---|
| Addison's disease with | Obesity |
| Hashimoto's | Slow healing |
| thyroiditis | |
| ↓ Pituitary reserve | |
| (occasionally) | |
| ↑ Glucocorticoid | |
| metabolism with | |
| $T_4$ therapy | |

signs and symptoms of hypothyroidism are listed in Table 6–9.) In mild to moderate cases the findings can be so subtle that the diagnosis may not be considered. Obesity and depression, which are common disorders, could appear to account for many of the findings in this disease. Even in the most severe cases, surgical conditions, especially if associated with metabolic derangements, could be assumed to account for fatigue, lethargy, and mental slowness. Consequently, the physician must keep the diagnosis in mind in order to make it.

(2) In addition to the physical appearance and history, the diagnosis might also be expected from a physiologic response that is inappropriate to the clinical setting. Patients with serious and painful surgical problems may be expected to have a rapid heart rate—a relative bradycardia may raise one's suspicion. Low or normal temperatures in patients with septic surgical conditions may also suggest the diagnosis, especially if other signs of hypothyroidism are present. Finally, one must be especially cautious with patients who have had prior diagnosis of hyperthyroidism or history of ablative therapy.

(3) There is probably no substitute for having seen several myxedematous patients to help suggest the diagnosis on subsequent occasions.

b. Laboratory diagnosis

The diagnosis of hypothyroidism can be confirmed by laboratory testing. Eighty-five per cent of cases will have a low $T_4$ value.[1, 15] When clinical suspicion is high but the screening $T_4$ test is within the low/normal range, an elevated thyroid-stimulating hormone (TSH) level usually will confirm the diagnosis. Secondary hypothyroidism (pituitary dysfunction), in which both $T_4$ and TSH levels are low, is uncommon but important to recognize. Pituitary dysfunction may produce life-threatening secondary adrenal insufficiency. Patients with this condition may be recognized by historical and physical evidence of lack of sex hormone effects. Laboratory tests should show gonadotropin or prolactin deficiency. If secondary hypothyroidism is diagnosed, adrenal response to stress should be evaluated. In emergency cases in which this assessment cannot be made, even the suspicion of inadequate adrenal

## TABLE 6–9. Symptomatology of Myxedema

| Symptom | Percentage of Cases* | Symptom | Percentage of Cases* |
|---|---|---|---|
| Weakness | 99 | Constipation | 61 |
| Dry skin | 97 | Gain in weight | 59 |
| Coarse skin | 97 | Loss of hair | 57 |
| Lethargy | 91 | Pallor of lips | 57 |
| Slow speech | 91 | Dyspnea | 55 |
| Edema of eyelids | 90 | Peripheral edema | 55 |
| Sensation of cold | 89 | Hoarseness or aphonia | 52 |
| Decreased sweating | 89 | Anorexia | 45 |
| Cold skin | 83 | Nervousness | 35 |
| Thick tongue | 82 | Menorrhagia | 32 |
| Edema of face | 79 | Palpitation | 31 |
| Coarseness of hair | 76 | Deafness | 30 |
| Pallor of skin | 67 | Precordial pain | 25 |
| Memory impairment | 66 | | |

From Ingbar SH, Woeber KA: The thyroid gland, in Williams RH (ed), Textbook of Endocrinology, 6th ed. Philadelphia, WB Saunders, 1981, p 213.
*Number of cases: 77 (64 women; 13 men).

function requires the administration of steroids during stress until further evaluation is possible[5, 15] (see Chapter 7). As a practical note, one should realize that the $T_3RU$ and the $T_3RIA$, which are helpful in diagnosing hyperthyroidism, may not be helpful in diagnosing hypothyroidism. Although the results of these tests are expected to be low, they may be normal in as many as 50 per cent of hypothyroid patients[16] (see Table 6–4).

## B. SURGICAL RISK FACTORS

Because thyroid function is responsible for the metabolic rate throughout the body, a deficiency affects virtually every organ system. In addition, a chronic deficiency can also lead to structural alterations, such as myxedematous infiltration of muscles[4] and enhanced atherosclerosis.[17] Some of the physiologic and structural effects of hypothyroidism that may adversely affect surgical risk have already been outlined (see Table 6–8). Although patients with mild to moderate hypothyroidism may not fare worse with surgery than do euthyroid patients,[18] the organ dysfunction and the potential for further deterioration make restoration of the euthyroid state imperative whenever possible.

1. Cardiovascular alterations in hypothyroidism

Significant cardiovascular abnormalities include a reduced cardiac contractility (which can be corrected by thyroid hormone replacement),[19] a low blood volume,[15] hypertension, and an above-average incidence of coronary atherosclerosis.[17] This combination of factors makes hypothyroid patients more susceptible to episodes of cardiac failure, hypotension, and resulting ischemic events. It is also noteworthy that elevated levels of creatine phosphokinase (CPK), lactic dehydrogenase (LDH) and serum glutamic oxaloacetic transaminase (SGOT)—but not serum glutemic pyruvic transaminase (SGPT)—found in hypothyroidism can cause confusion in the evaluation of possible cardiac events.[4, 20] The myocardial isoenzyme of CPK (MB fraction) is not elevated in hypothyroidism and therefore is helpful in evaluating possible myocardial events.[21] Pericardial and pleural effusions may be seen in hypothyroid patients but are only rarely the cause of compromised organ function.[4]

2. Pulmonary alterations in hypothyroidism

Pulmonary function is compromised in hypothyroid patients. Alveolar hypoventilation can result from various causes:

   a. A reduced responsiveness of the respiratory center to hypoxia and, in more profound cases, hypercapnia[22, 23]
   b. An increased susceptibility to sedatives[24]
   c. Myxedematous infiltration of respiratory muscles[4]
   d. Reduced compliance, secondary to obesity

     When other factors known to compromise pulmonary function are added, such as abdominal or thoracic surgery and pre-existing lung disease, the risk of ventilatory insufficiency may be quite high.

3. Drug sensitivity

     The lower rate of drug metabolism,[25] along with the extreme sensitivity to CNS depressants,[26] makes it imperative that the consultant point out the need for reduced doses of both sedatives and narcotics.

## C. SURGICAL MANAGEMENT OF THE HYPOTHYROID PATIENT

     Because of the compromise in the various organ systems, elective surgery should not be undertaken until the hypothyroid state has been corrected. With the exception of myxedema coma, the replacement of thyroid hormone is not an emergency.[4] Additionally, hypothyroid patients are extremely sensitive to the affects of thyroid hormone.[4] Therefore, replacement should begin with modest doses and should be increased gradually over two to four weeks as the clinical setting indicates. In the majority of cases in which hypothyroidism is primary, the clinician can monitor the TSH level to complement his or her clinical impression of the patient's return to the euthyroid state. In the young, medically stable patient, therapy should be initiated with 25 to 50 μg of levothyroxine daily and the dose increased by 25 μg at intervals of two weeks until the full replacement dosage is attained (100 to 200 μg/day). In older patients who are less medically stable, therapy should be initiated with 25 μg/day and raised by 12.5 to 25 μg every two to four weeks, depending on the clinical setting. In patients with serious underlying cardiac disease and angina pectoris, replacement therapy must proceed extremely gradually. If congestive heart failure is not present, the use of propranolol or other beta blocking agents may be appropriate during the replacement phase.

## D. MYXEDEMA COMA

     Myxedema coma is the most serious form of hypothyroidism and usually occurs in patients with severe, long-standing thyroid hormone deficiency.[4] The syndrome itself is rare, but clinical conditions mimicking this entity are common. Because the mortality is approximately 50 per cent even for appropriately treated patients, the clinician cannot ignore even the possibility of myxedema coma.[27] Although it may occur in both young and old, as well as in both males and females, it is most commonly seen in women older than age 50 and usually during the winter. Virtually all patients who develop coma have a precipitating cause, the most common of which is infection.[28] Although pneumonia is the most common precipitating infection, a surgical catastrophe or the surgical procedure itself may be the precipitating event that brings the patient to the attention of the consulting internist. Other precipitating factors include myocardial infarction, congestive heart failure, and drugs, primarily sedatives, narcotics, and tranquilizers. Even though infections tend to raise the temperature, this entity usually is accompanied by a subnormal temperature, the depth of which may not be appreciated with the usual clinical thermometer, which goes to only 94°F. Other clinical features include bradycardia, hypotension, and delayed or absent deep tendon reflexes. Hypoventilation with carbon dioxide retention is also a common clinical feature.

1. Differential diagnosis of myxedema coma

    Although myxedema coma is rare, other conditions, which are more common, may be difficult to distinguish from this entity at their presentation. One of these conditions is obesity in patients who may have sustained a brain stem infarction, a drug overdose, or cold exposure, all of which could result in hypothermia, hypotension, and bradycardia.[4, 29]

2. Therapy of myxedema coma

    Because of the high mortality in myxedema coma,[15] therapy must begin immediately, before the results of the thyroid function tests are known.

    a. Thyroid hormone

        Hormone replacement is given as a single IV dose of 400 to 500 μg of levothyroxine, which serves to rapidly replete the hormone pool and may be followed by clinical improvement within 24 hours.[4] Although the adequacy of levothyroxine therapy in these cases is questionable, owing to the possible inhibition of peripheral conversion to triiodothyronine in these severely ill patients, insufficient data exist to recommend an alternative therapy.

    b. Glucocorticoids

        It is also important that hydrocortisone be given IV in doses of 50 to 100 mg every eight hours. This is to allow for the possibility that the increased metabolic rate induced by thyroid hormone replacement might temporily cause the catabolism of glucocorticoids to exceed the adrenal synthetic capacity. It also will protect against those rare cases in which hypothyroidism is secondary to pituitary failure and therefore associated with secondary adrenal insufficiency.

c. Additional supportive therapy

While awaiting the laboratory results, the patient should be checked for hypoglycemia and glucose adminstered. Care must be taken in the administration of IV fluids to avoid exacerbating hyponatremia, commonly seen with hypothyroidism. External rewarming must be limited in order to avoid peripheral vascular collapse. Respiratory support should be initiated when appropriate. Finally, one should not forget to seek and treat a precipitating cause or underlying disease aggressively.

## REFERENCES

1. Aubid J, Larsen PR: Triiodothyroine and thyroxine in hyperthyroidism: Comparison of the acute changes during therapy with antithyroid agents. J Clin Invest 54:201, 1974.
2. Nusynowitz ML, Young RL: Thyroid dysfunction in the ailing, aging and aberrant (editorial). JAMA 242:275, 1979.
3. Williams RH: Thiouracil treatment of thyrotoxicosis, in The results of prolonged treatment. J Clin Endocrinol 6:1, 1946.
4. Ingbar SH, Woeber KA: The thyroid gland, in Williams RH (ed): Textbook of Endocrinology, 6th ed. Philadelphia, WB Saunders, 1981, p 209.
5. Hoffenberg R: Thyroid emergencies. Clin Endocrinol Metab 9:503, 1980.
6. Caswell HT, Marks AD, Channick BJ: Propranolol for the preoperative preparation of patients with thyrotoxicosis. Surg Gynecol Obstet 146:908, 1978.
7. Eriksson M, Rubenfeld S, Garger A, et al: Propranolol does not prevent thyroid storm. N Engl J Med 296:263, 1977.
8. Zonszein J, Santangelo RP, Makin JF, et al: Propranolol therapy in thyrotoxicosis: A review of 84 patients undergoing surgery. Am J Med 66:411, 1979.
9. Lee TC, Coffey RJ, Mackin J, et al: The use of propranolol in the surgical treatment of thyrotoxic patients. Ann Surg 177:643, 1973.
10. Gladstone GR, Hosdof A, Gersony WM: Propranolol administration during pregnancy: Effects on the fetus. J Pediatr 86:962–964, 1975.
11. Tunstall ME: The effect of propranolol on the onset of breathing at birth. Br J Anaesth 41:792, 1969.

12. McArthur JW, Rawson RW, Means JH, et al: Thyrotoxic crisis. JAMA 134:868, 1947.

13. Feek CM, Sowers SA, Irvine WJ: Combination of potassium iodide and propranolol in preparation of patients with Graves' disease for thyroid surgery. N Engl J Med 302:883, 1980.

14. Hershman JM: The treatment of hyperthyroidism. Ann Intern Med 64:1306, 1966.

15. Das KC, Mukhergee M, Sarkar TK, et al: Erythropoiesis and erythropoietin in hypo- and hyperthyroidism. J Clin Endocrinol Metab 41:211, 1975.

16. Brown J, Chopra IJ, Cornell JS, et al: Thyroid physiology in health and disease. Ann Intern Med 81:68, 1964.

17. VanHaelst L, Neve PE, Shailly M, Bastenie PA: Coronary artery disease in hypothyroidism. Lancet 2:800, 1967.

18. Molitch ME: Endocrinology, in Molitch ME (ed): Management of Medical Problems in Surgical Patients. Philadelphia, FA Davis, 1982, p 173.

19. Crowley WF Jr, Ridgeway EC, Bough EW, et al: Noninvasive evaluation of cardiac function in hypothyroidism. N Engl J Med 296:1, 1977.

20. Aber CP, Nobel RL, Thompson GS, et al: Serum lactic dehydrogenase isoenzymes in "myxedema heart disease." Br Heart J 27:663, 1966.

21. Goldman J, Matz R, Mortimer R, et al: High elevations of creatinine phosphokinase in hypothyroidism, in Isoenzyme analysis. JAMA 27:325, 1977.

22. Massumi RA, Winnacker JL: Severe depression of the respiratory center in myxedema. Am J Med 36:876, 1964.

23. Zwillich ZW, Pierson DJ, Hofeldt FD, et al: Ventilatory control in myxedema and hypothyroidism. N Engl J Med 292:62, 1975.

24. Kim JM, Hackman L: Anesthesia for untreated hyperthyroidism: Report of three cases. Anesth Analg 56:299, 1977.

25. Eichelbaum M, Bodem G, Gugler R, et al: Influence of thyroid status of plasma half-life of antipyrine in man. N Engl J Med 290:1040, 1974.

26. Royce PC: Severely impaired consciousness in myxedema—A review. Am J Med Sci 261:6, 1971.

27. Nicoloff JF: Myxedema coma. Pharmacol Ther 1:161, 1976.

28. Katz B, Russel S: Myxedema shock and coma: Seven survival cases. Arch Intern Med 108:129, 1961.

29. Reuler JB: Hypothermia: Pathophysiology, clinical settings, and management. Ann Intern Med 89:519, 1978.

# 7

# ADRENAL DYSFUNCTION AND STEROID USE

## I. PREOPERATIVE EVALUATION

### A. PURPOSE

The real problem in evaluating preoperative patients comes not in the management of adrenal insufficiency, but in identifying those patients who need supplemental steroids. Patients with frank adrenal insufficiency may not be recognized if signs and symptoms are attributed to overwhelming illness. It is even more difficult to identify the patient with adequate basal cortisol secretion but inadequate adrenal reserves, because, in these patients, the adrenal cortex works to capacity simply to maintain basal cortisol requirements. Although such levels are adequate for daily activity, without any reserve they cannot be increased as required during stress. Because the maximal adrenal output can meet basal requirements in these patients, there are no symptoms to arouse suspicion.

### B. CLINICAL ASSESSMENT

1. History and physical examination

Because clinical clues and problems facing the clinician depend, to some degree, on the site of dysfunction, glucocorticoid deficiency should be separated into three types and dealt with accordingly:

a. Primary dysfunction at the level of the adrenal gland. A suggestive history usually includes complaints of weakness, weight loss, anorexia, and fatigue. In some cases such historical factors as disseminated tuberculosis, sarcoidosis, and poor response to stress in the past may be important. Physical findings, such as hypotension and hyperpigmentation, also may be significant clues.

  b. Secondary adrenal insufficiency. Where there is pituitary disease, the physician must be alert for other pituitary hormone deficiencies.
  c. Adrenal suppression owing to the administration of exogenous steroid. History of recent exogenous steroid use is, of course, most important. Suspicion may otherwise be aroused by a cushingoid appearance or evidence of systemic disease frequently treated with steroids.

  Because of the differences in these clinical presentations, they are discussed individually and in greater detail later.
2. Laboratory assessment. Determining the ability of the adrenal gland to respond to maximum stress during surgery is the goal of evaluation. See the detailed discussion below.

## II. SURGICAL RISK FACTORS

Adrenocortical deficiency has frequently been reported as being associated with cardiovascular collapse during stress and surgery.[1, 2] Some reports of cardiovascular collapse from adrenal deficiency secondary to exogenous steroid administration have been questioned on grounds of inadequate documentation.[3, 4] Other reports, even though clearly showing low cortisol levels at the time of collapse, have just as clearly shown that similar patients undergoing similar surgery develop no cardiovascular instability despite even lower cortisol levels.[5, 6] Because of this conflicting information and the great variety of possible surgical situations, one cannot define precisely a patient's risk.

However, despite the scientific questions that might be raised, the volume of medical literature describing vascular collapse in adrenal deficiency forces the practicing physician to accept this as fact.[6] Corticosteroid "coverage" has become a standard practice when treating patients with even suspected adrenal deficiency who undergo surgery.

## III. PRIMARY ADRENAL FAILURE

### A. ETIOLOGY OF PRIMARY ADRENAL FAILURE

Primary adrenal failure results from surgical ablation or destruction of the adrenal glands by one of the pathologic processes listed in Table 7–1.

**TABLE 7–1. Pathologic Causes of Primary Adrenal Failure**

Idiopathic atrophy
  Autoimmune adrenalitis
Infectious diseases
  Tuberculosis, bacteremia, fungal diseases
Infiltrative diseases
  Amyloidosis, carcinoma, hemorrhage, infarction

Modified from Williams G, Dluhy R, Thorn G: Dieases of the adrenal cortex, in Thorn G, et al (eds.): Harrison's Principles of Internal Medicine, 8th ed. New York, McGraw-Hill, 1976, p 547.

## B. SYMPTOMS OF PRIMARY ADRENAL FAILURE

Virtually all patients with chronic primary adrenal failure will have weakness, weight loss, and anorexia, as shown in Table 7–2. Unfortunately, these symptoms are nonspecific and may be attributed to another illness. Increased dermal pigmentation resulting from melanocyte stimulation by adrenocorticotropic hormone (ACTH) is common but may be subtle. The increased pigment should be most prominent in the skin folds.

## C. ALDOSTERONE DEFICIENCY ASSOCIATED WITH PRIMARY FAILURE

In addition to low cortisol levels, aldosterone deficiency is also present, preventing the kidneys from preserving sodium at the same time that anorexia and vomiting have reduced oral intake. The combination of these factors leads to a depletion of extracellular fluid volume, with a reduction

**TABLE 7–2. Symptoms of Chronic Primary Adrenocortical Insufficiency**

| Clinical Feature | Per Cent |
| --- | --- |
| Weakness and fatigue | 100 |
| Weight loss | 100 |
| Anorexia | 100 |
| Hyperpigmentation | 92 |
| Hypotension | 88 |
| Gastrointestinal symptoms | 56 |
| Salt craving | 19 |
| Postural symptoms | 12 |

From Baxter JD, Blake TJ: The adrenal cortex, in Felig P, et al (eds.): Endocrinology and Metabolism. New York, McGraw-Hill, 1981, p 453.

in blood pressure as well as cardiac output. This development may hasten the onset of peripheral vascular collapse during exposure to stress. When treating a patient with clinical deterioration resulting from primary adrenal deficiency, the replacement of sodium and fluid volume is as critical as the administration of the deficient hormones. Table 7–3 shows the clinical manifestation of cortisol and aldosterone deficiencies.

## D. ACUTE ADRENAL CRISIS

Findings in acute adrenal crisis are similar to those in the chronic state except for their fulminant nature. The setting, however, is likely to be one of sudden stress, such as the development of a surgical condition (e.g., appendicitis). Some findings in patients with adrenal crisis are noted in Table 7–4.

Although the setting may be one with symptoms of chronic adrenal deficiency with sudden crisis, it is much more likely that basal cortisol secretion will prevent symptoms before the onset of surgical stress. Because most of the signs listed in Table 7–4 could be attributed to an acute surgical disease, adrenal insufficiency may not be suspected. The physician should be especially suspicious in surgical cases with pro-

**TABLE 7–3. Clinical Manifestations of Cortisol and Aldosterone Deficiency**

| Cortisol Deficiency | Aldosterone Deficiency |
|---|---|
| Loss of appetite | Inability of distal tubule to conserve sodium |
| Loss of vigor | |
| Inability to maintain normal glucose with fasting | Inability to normally excrete potassium and hydrogen |
| Inability to excrete free water | Extracellular fluid depletion |
| Occasional dilutional hyponatremia | Intravascular volume depletion |
| Inability to withstand stress | Supine or orthostatic hypotension |
| Shock | Occasional hyponatremia |
| Exaggerated fever | Occasional hyperkalemia |
| Pigmentation | Occasional prerenal azotemia |
| | Occasional acidosis |

From Byyny RL: Management of adrenal insufficiency during stress or surgery. Unpublished.

TABLE 7–4. Clinical Features of Adrenal Crisis

| Finding | No. Abnormal / No. Observations | % Abnormal Findings |
|---|---|---|
| Temperature of 103° F or higher | 77/110 | 70 |
| Shock (systolic BP 80 or less) | 25/110 | 23 |
| Serum sodium reduced (130 mEq/L or less) | 43/109 | 39 |
| Hemoconcentration (Hct greater than 45%) | 23/73 | 32 |
| Nitrogen retention (BUN greater than 25) | 12/66 | 18 |
| Serum potassium elevated (6 mEq/L or more) | 13/72 | 18 |
| Hypoglycemia (blood sugar less than 70 mg/100 ml) | 8/61 | 13 |

From Knowlton AI: Addison's disease, in Christy NR (ed.): The Human Adrenal Cortex. New York, Harper & Row, 1971, p 329.

longed or unexplained fever and shock. Failure to suspect this diagnosis may lead to death from a preventable cause.

# IV. SECONDARY ADRENAL FAILURE

## A. ASSOCIATED PITUITARY HORMONE DEFICIENCIES

Adrenal insufficiency secondary to pituitary dysfunction or iatrogenic suppression will differ slightly from primary cases. Most symptoms and signs are the same, but in pituitary disease associated endocrine abnormalities may be present, such as hypothyroidism, diabetes insipidus, and sex steroid deficiencies. In some cases the hypothyroidism is the most prominent finding. As discussed in Chapter 6, corticosteroid coverage should be administered along with thyroid hormone in newly discovered cases of hypothyroidism until the functional status of the Hypothalamic-Pituitary-Adrenal (HPA) system can be determined.

## B. DERMAL PIGMENTATION AND ALDOSTERONE DEFICIENCY

Dermal pigmentation will not be present in either iatrogenic or secondary adrenal insufficiency, since ACTH production is low in both. Despite the fact that mineralocorticoid production is influenced to some degree by ACTH, the findings of aldosterone deficiency will not be present, as its primary regulation occurs through the undisturbed renin-angiotensin system. It is important to note, however, that even without the degree of extracellular volume depletion that would be expected from aldosterone deficiency, cardiovascular collapse does occur from cortisol deficiency alone.

# V. IATROGENIC ADRENAL DEFICIENCY

It is generally accepted that the most common cause of adrenal insufficiency is the therapeutic administration of steroids.[11] However, the number of patients with actual adrenal suppression is small compared with the number of patients who are treated with steroids. The management of adrenal insufficiency is not difficult; the real problem is deciding which patients actually need steroid coverage.

## A. EXPERIMENTAL DATA ON ADRENAL SUPPRESSION WITH CORTICOSTEROIDS—EFFECT OF DOSE, FREQUENCY, TIMING, AND DURATION

Biochemical evidence of adrenal suppression has been known to relate to glucocorticoid dose,[12] frequency,[13] timing,[14] duration of therapy,[15] route of administration,[16] and duration of action of the agent used.[17] Doses of prednisone of less than 40 mg given once daily in the morning for five to seven days usually will not cause adrenal suppression.[11, 18, 19] However, short courses of larger doses or longer courses of lower doses may produce suppression.[11] Alternate-day therapy with 40 mg of prednisone does not cause significant suppression, even with long-term administration.[11, 13]

1. Duration

Myles and associates[20] found that long-term (8 to 40 months') administration of 5 to 10 mg of prednisolone to 12 patients with rheumatoid arthritis produced no HPA suppression when given as single morning doses.

2. Timing and frequency

Of seven patients given amounts of prednisolone equal to those in the study just described, except twice daily, three showed HPA suppression.[20]

3. Dose and frequency

Klinefelter and co-workers[21] evaluated the response to ACTH in 42 patients taking a single daily dose of prednisone from 1 to 19 years. They found that all patients taking 7.5 mg or less of prednisone once daily had a normal response to ACTH. This was true even if they took their dose at night. For patients in the 10-to-12.5-mg range, 33 per cent had a blunted response; of patients taking 15 mg, 47 per cent showed a blunted response. As long as the single-dose regimen was maintained, complete suppression was avoided until the 20-mg dose was reached.

4. Preparation

   Some authors have shown that the use of longer-acting preparations, especially at night, can significantly suppress the 17-hydroxycorticosteroid (17-OHCS) output.[17, 21, 22]

5. Minimum time to suppression

   Christy and associates[19] demonstrated an impaired response to ACTH in one patient on 30 mg of prednisone for five days and in two patients on 20 mg of prednisone for seven days. Abnormal responses to ACTH have been found after three days of 100 mg of cortisol daily.[23]

## B. TIME COURSE OF ADRENAL RECOVERY

1. Recovery after long-term suppression

   The classic study by Graber and co-workers[24] provides a background for assessing HPA recovery. These investigators followed eight patients with Cushing's syndrome who had a unilateral adrenocortical tumor removed at surgery, and six patients who had taken physiologic doses of glucocorticoids for 1 to 10 years. Plasma 17-OHCS, plasma ACTH, and the adrenal response to ACTH were measured. Results are shown in Table 7–5.

**TABLE 7–5. Test Results After Steroid Withdrawal**

| Time Lapse (months) | Plasma 17-OHCS | Plasma ACTH | Adrenal Response to ACTH |
|---|---|---|---|
| 1 | Low* | Low | Low |
| 2–5 | Low | High† | Low |
| 3–9 | Normal | Normal | Low |
| 9 | Normal | Normal | Normal |

*In this phase the patients had subjective manifestations of adrenal insufficiency.
†Qualitatively normal diurnal rhythm of plasma concentration during this phase.
Modified from Graber A, Ney R, Nicholson W, et al: Natural history of pituitary-adrenal recovery following long-term suppression with corticosteroids. J Clin Endocrinol Metab 25:11, 1965.

These authors found that during the first month, baseline output of 17-OHCS was low, ACTH was low, and the patients had symptoms of adrenal insufficiency. From two to five months, baseline 17-OHCS were normal, plasma ACTH was high, and the adrenal response to ACTH stimulation was still low. From six to nine months, baseline 17-OHCS and ACTH were normal, but there was still a subnormal adrenal response to ACTH stimulation. It was not until more than nine months had passed that all parameters were normal. This suggests that pituitary output of ACTH returns first, with supranormal levels resulting from poor adrenal function. In the six-to-nine-month period, although ACTH and 17-OHCS were normal, a poor response to ACTH stimulation still indicated impaired adrenal reserve.

2. Conclusions on recovery

Other reports give similar periods of adrenal recovery after glucocorticoid therapy.[3, 18] What does this mean with regard to predicting recovery? After reviewing the data, Axelrod concludes: "If the glucocorticoid is given in pharmacologic doses for a period of more than one to four weeks, patients undergoing general anesthesia or other metabolic stressful experiences should be suspected of having HPA suppression up to one year after the termination of therapy."[3]

## C. JUDGING ADRENAL RESERVE: THE ACTH STIMULATION TEST

When the available information is inadequate to assess the likelihood of adrenal suppression, either of two courses can be taken. The patient may be assumed to have inadequate adrenal reserves and steroids are empirically administered, or the adrenal reserve can be measured by an ACTH stimulation test (described later). Numerous studies have found that patients with a normal response to an ACTH stimulation test showed an adequate adrenal response during surgery and had no episodes of cardiovascular collapse.[6, 8] Although the administration of a steroid cover in all questionable cases is the simplest procedure, there is a possibility of needlessly impairing wound healing and increasing susceptibility to infection.[3, 25] This becomes even more of a concern if postoperative complications require that the empirical steroid therapy continue longer than originally planned. In surgical emergencies, when an ACTH stimulation test is impractical, a random cortisol can be obtained during stress and steroids administered. A value of 22 μg/dl or greater is generally considered to indicate normal pituitary adrenal responsiveness and no further therapy is needed.[11] However, doubts about the safety of even this level of responsiveness have been raised (see VIB below).

## VI. HOW MUCH GLUCOCORTICOID IS REQUIRED?

If steroid coverage is to be given, it is necessary to know how much should be given and for what period of time to prevent adrenal crisis during surgical stress. Because there is no way of knowing how much steroid the body needs for an individual situation, one assumes that providing steroid coverage equal to the maximal stimulated adrenal output of normal individuals would give adequate coverage. This dose should be administered in such a way as to provide serum cortisol levels equal to levels found in normal individuals undergoing surgery. Levels should be maintained above the highest levels that have been found in patients who have undergone vascular collapse susequently reversed by steroid administration.

### A. MAXIMAL STIMULATED CORTISOL OUTPUT OF NORMALS

Maximal cortisol output with ACTH stimulation has been reported to range from 116 to 185 mg daily.[11, 26] Under maximal stress, cortisol production can reach 200 to 500 mg/day.[11, 27] Given these values, replacement doses of hydrocortisone of 300 to 400 mg/day are generally used during severe stress. Plumpton and associates[28] measured cortisol levels in 20 patients undergoing major surgery and 20 patients undergoing minor surgery. The mean plasma cortisol peak for major surgery was 47 μg/dl (range 22 to 75), with all patients' cortisol levels returning to baseline within 72 hours. The mean peak for minor surgery was 28 μg/dl (range 10 to 44), and all levels returned to baseline within 24 hours.

### B. SPECIAL CONSIDERATIONS

Complicating these data somewhat are reports by both Mattingly and Tyler[29] and Oyama,[5] who have documented cardiovascular collapse apparently responsive to steroids when cortisol levels were above 20 μg/dl. Therefore, it becomes important to be sure that the preparation used and route of administration give adequate serum levels.

## C. EFFECT ON DOSE PREPARATION AND ROUTE

Plumpton and co-workers[30] measured plasma cortisol levels with administration of intramuscular cortisone acetate and IV and IM hydrocortisone hemisuccinate. Cortisone acetate was given as 100 mg IM the night before surgery, 100 mg IM b.i.d. the day of surgery and the following postoperative day, and then on a tapering oral schedule. Hydrocortisone hemisuccinate (100 mg) was given IM every six hours for three days from the time of premedication, or, alternatively, 100 mg IV as a single dose with the induction of anesthesia. Figures 7–1 to 7–3 show the resulting serum levels.

One hundred milligrams of hydrocortisone given IM provided a peak level of 80 μg/dl, which fell to 30 μg/dl at six hours. When given IV, the same dose gave peak cortisol levels of over 150 μg/dl but the level fell to 33 μg/dl at four hours and to 18 μg/dl at six hours. Cortisone acetate, once recommended as an appropriate drug for steroid cover,[32] did not provide levels in the 20 μg/dl range until approximately eight hours after the initiation of surgery.[30] This is less than one half the mean found in normals in response to major surgical stress. Because of these low levels and the

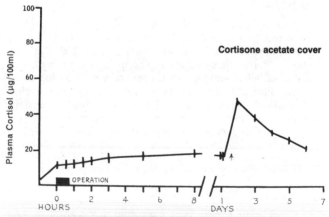

**Figure 7–1.** Plasma cortisol levels in five currently steroid-treated patients having minor surgery under cortisone acetate cover. Mean values and standard errors are shown. The arrow shows the time of changing from intramuscular to oral cover. (From Plumpton FS, Besser GM, Cole PV: Corticosteroid treatment and surgery. 2. The management of steroid cover. Anesthesia 24:13, 1969.)

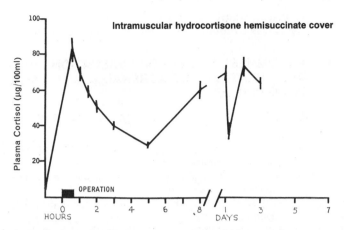

**Figure 7–2.** Plasma cortisol levels in ten currently steroid-treated patients having minor surgery under intramuscular hydrocortisone hemisuccinate cover. Mean values and standard errors are shown. (From Plumpton FS, Besser GM, Cole PV: Corticosteroid treatment and surgery. 2. The management of steroid cover. Anesthesia 24:13, 1969.)

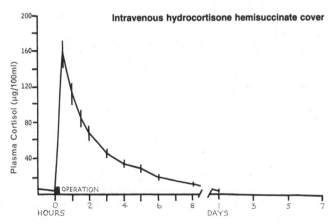

**Figure 7–3.** Plasma cortisol levels in five currently steroid-treated patients having minor surgery under intravenous hydrocortisone hemisuccinate cover (100 mg with the induction of anesthesia). Mean values and standard errors are shown. Note that the vertical scale has been halved in comparison with Figures 7–1 and 7–2. (From Plumpton FS, Besser GM, Cole PV: Corticosteroid treatment and surgery. 2. The management of steroid cover. Anesthesia 24:13, 1969.)

fact that operative shock has been reported in patients covered with cortisone acetate,[31] its use *is not recommended*!

## VII. RECOMMENDATIONS FOR EVALUATION AND TREATMENT OF ADRENAL INSUFFICIENCY

### A. CLINICAL SUSPICION OF ADRENAL DEFICIENCY

1. Patients should be suspected of having adrenal deficiency if they have taken steroids in any of the following schedules in the past year:
   a. More than 7.5 mg of prednisone in a single daily dose longer than one month
   b. Any steroid in divided doses for longer than five to seven days
   c. Long-acting preparations (dexamethasone or beta-methasone) for longer than five to seven days
   d. More than 20 mg of prednisone daily (in single or divided doses) for longer than five to seven days.
   One should also suspect adrenal deficiency if:
   e. Patient has a cushingoid appearance
   f. Patient has taken daily steroid doses for longer than one week but does not know the dose
   g. Patient is in unexplained or prolonged shock or has a fever.
2. Patients are unlikely to have an adrenal deficiency if:
   a. They have taken 40 mg of prednisone or less on an alternate-day schedule only
   b. They have taken ACTH in any schedule for less than one year
   c. They have used topical or inhalant steroids. (Such steroids can cause adrenal suppression, but this rarely occurs.)
3. ACTH stimulation test
   If the diagnosis of adrenal deficiency is suspected and the patient is stable, one may either do an ACTH stimulation test (see Table 7–6), in which a normal result excludes any need for steroid coverage, or give replacement doses of steroids.

### B. PROCEDURE FOR GLUCOCORTICOID REPLACEMENT

1. Major elective surgery
   a. Hydrocortisone sodium succinate 100 mg IM or IV every 6 hours for 24 hours, to start with preoperative

TABLE 7-6. ACTH Stimulation Test

| Agent | Basal Plasma Cortisol (μg/dl) | Cortisol 30–60 min After Stimulation (μg/dl) | Minimum Increment 30–60 min After Stimulation (μg/dl) |
|---|---|---|---|
| Cosyntropin (synthetic ACTH) 250 μg IM or IV | Greater than 5 | Greater than 18 | Greater than 7 |

medication. Use the IV route in the presence of tissue hypoperfusion.

b. Provide adequate fluid glucose and electrolytes.

c. Reduce hydrocortisone by 50 per cent daily, beginning on first postoperative day until either maintenance dosage of hydrocortisone (20 mg in A.M., 10 mg in P.M.) or equivalent steroid is reached, or preoperative steroid regimen is resumed, for example:

First postoperative day: hydrocortisone 50 mg IV or IM q6

Second postoperative day: hydrocortisone 25 mg IV or IM q6

Third postoperative day: hydrocortisone 25 mg IV or IM q12

Fourth postoperative day: hydrocortisone 20 mg in A.M., 10 mg in P.M., parenterally or PO when tolerated.

If patient is on higher-than-normal maintenance dosage of steroid before surgery (for condition other than adrenal insufficiency), postoperative steroid dosage should be maintained when the equivalent level of hydrocortisone is reached.

d. In patients with primary adrenal insufficiency, fludrocortisone, 0.1 mg daily, must be added to provide sufficient mineralocorticoid activity when the dose of hydrocortosone is 100 mg or less per day.

e. If the patient has complications or manifests symptoms of adrenal deficiency during tapering, increase the dose.

2. Elective minor procedures
   a. Hydrocortisone sodium succinate 100 mg IM or IV every 6 hours for 24 hours, beginning with premedication.
   b. Reduce hydrocortisone to 20 mg A.M., 10 mg P.M., or resume preoperative steroid regimen.

3. Short procedures
   a. A single IM or IV dose of hydrocortisone sodium succinate, 100 mg, should be given with premedication and an extra dose of 20 mg given orally that evening.
   b. Resume prior steroid therapy on the following day.

4. Emergency evaluation and treatment
   If the diagnosis is suspected in an emergency that demands empiric therapy, a combination diagnostic and therapeutic approach should be used.
   a. Obtain blood for cortisol and ACTH determination (as well as electrolyte, creatinine, BUN). Both values

will be low in hypothalamic pituitary disease, but ACTH will be elevated in primary adrenal disease.

b. Start a rapid infusion of dextrose and normal saline or colloid to correct volume deficit.

c. Give cosyntropin (synthetic ACTH) 250 μg IM or IV (preferred over animal ACTH, which has higher incidence of allergic reactions).

d. At same time, give dexamethasone phosphate 4 mg IV (dexamethasone will not interfere with the cortisol assay or the adrenal's response to ACTH).

e. Draw blood for evaluation of cortisol one hour after administration of cosyntropin or ACTH.

f. Continue dexamethasone phosphate 4 mg IM or IV q6 for at least 24 hours and then taper, based on results of test.

g. As noted in Table 7–6, minimum accepted values for the ACTH stimulation test are a basal cortisol of greater than 5 μg/dl and an increment of greater than 7 μg/dl, with actual level over 18 μg/dl. In a stressed patient, basal cortisol is expected to be considerably higher than 5 μg/dl and response should be close to a doubling of basal value. In patients with primary adrenal disease, little response is seen; in patients with secondary disease, a response is present, although subnormal. It is important to perform this test in suspected adrenal insufficiency so that steroid administration can be stopped if adrenal responsiveness is normal (the clinical impression of adrenal insufficiency is in error). However, the ACTH stimulation test is only a screening test and an abnormal test requires more extensive and prolonged testing of the HPA areas for confirmation, once the patient is stable.

## REFERENCES

1. Salassa R, Bennett W, Keating F, Sprague R: Postoperative adrenal cortical insufficiency: Occurrence in patients previously treated with cortisone. JAMA *152*:1509, 1953.
2. Lewis L, Robinson R, Yee J, et al: Fatal adrenal cortical insufficiency precipitated by surgery during prolonged continuous cortisone treatment. Ann Intern Med *39*:116, 1953.
3. Axelrod L: Glucocorticoid therapy. Medicine *55*:39, 1976.
4. Slaney G, Brooke B: Postoperative collapse due to adrenal insufficiency following cortisone therapy. Lancet *1*:1167, 1957.

5. Oyama T: Hazards of steroids in association with anesthesia. Can Anaesth Soc J *16*:361, 1969.

6. Jason MK, Freeman PA, Boyle JA: Studies of the rise in plasma 11-hydroxycorticosteroids (11-OHCS) in corticosteroid-treated patients with rheumatoid arthritis during surgery: Correlations with the functional integrity of the hypothalamus-adrenal axis. *37*:407, 1968.

7. Sampson PA, Winstone NE, Brooke BN: Adrenal function in surgical patients after steroid therapy. Lancet *2*:322, 1962.

8. Sampson PA, Brooke BN, Winstone NE: Biochemical conformation of collapse due to adrenal failure. Lancet *1*:1377, 1961.

9. Allanby KD: Deaths associated with steroid hormone therapy: An analysis of 18 cases. Lancet *1*:1104, 1957.

10. Fraser LG, Preuse FS, Bigford WD: Adrenal atrophy and irreversible shock associated with cortisone therapy. JAMA *149*:1542, 1952.

11. Byyny RL: Preventing adrenal insufficiency during surgery. Postgrad Med *67*:219, 1980.

12. Donald RA: Dexamethasone suppression of the plasma corticosterone response to stress in the rat. J Physiol *182*:603, 1966.

13. Ackerman GL, Nolan CM: Adrenocortical responsiveness after alternate day corticosteroid therapy. N Engl J Med *278*:405, 1968.

14. Nicholas T, Nugent LA, Tyler FH: Diurnal variation and suppression of adrenal function by glucocorticoids. J Clin Endocrinol Metab *25*:343, 1965.

15. Treadwell BLJ, Savage D, Sever ED, et al: Pituitary adrenal function during corticosteroid therapy. Lancet *1*:355, 1963.

16. Maberly DJ, Gibson GJ, Butler AG: Recovery of adrenal function after substitution of beclomethasone dipropionate for oral corticosteroids. Br Med J *1*:778, 1973.

17. Rabhan NB: Pituitary-adrenal suppression and Cushing's syndrome after intermittent dexamethasone therapy. Ann Intern Med *69*:1141, 1968.

18. Livanou T, et al: Recovery of hypothalamopituitary-adrenal function after corticosteroid therapy. Lancet *2*:856, 1967.

19. Christy NP, Wallace EZ, Jailer JW: Comparative effects of prednisone and cortisone in suppressing the response of the adrenal cortex to exogenous adrenocorticotropin. J Clin Endocrinol Metab *16*:1059, 1956.

20. Myles A, Schiller L, Glass D, Daly J: Single daily dose corticosteroid treatment. Ann Rheum Dis *35*:73, 1976.

21. Klinefelter H, Winkenwerder W, Bledsoe T: Single daily dose prednisone therapy. JAMA *241*:2721, 1979.

22. Martin MM, Gaboardi F, Podolsky S, et al: Intermittent steroid therapy. N Engl J Med *279*:273, 1968.

23. Plager JE, Cushman P: Suppression of the pituitary—ACTH response in man by administration of ACTH or cortisol. J Clin Endocrinol Metab *22*:147, 1962.

24. Graber A, Ney R, Nicholson W, et al: Natural history of pituitary-adrenal recovery following long-term suppression with corticosteroids. J Clin Endocrinol Metab *25*:11, 1965.

25. Speckart PF, Nicoloff JT, Bethune JE: Screening for adrenocortical insufficiency with cosyntropin (synthetic ACTH). Arch Intern Med *128*:761, 1971.
26. Goldman DR: The surgical patient on steroids. *In* Medical Care of the Surgical Patient. Philadelphia, JB Lippincott, 1982.
27. Baxter JD, Blake TJ: The adrenal cortex, in Felig P, et al (eds): Endocrinology and Metabolism. New York, McGraw-Hill, 1981.
28. Plumpton EJ, Besser GM, Cole PV: Corticosteroid treatment and surgery: 1. An investigation of the indications for steroid cover. Anesthesia *24*:3, 1969.
29. Mattingly D, Tyler C: Plasma 11-hydroxycorticoid levels in surgical stress. Proc Roy Soc Med *58*:1010, 1965.
30. Plumpton FS, Besser GM, Cole PV: Corticosteroid treatment and surgery: 2. The management of steroid cover. Anesthesia *24*:13, 1969.
31. Bayliss RI: Surgical collapse during and after corticosteroid therapy. Br Med J *2*:935, 1958.

# 8

# CALCIUM METABOLISM

## I. HYPERCALCEMIA

### A. PREOPERATIVE EVALUATION

1. Purpose

   The hypercalcemic patient who is scheduled for surgery should be fully evaluated whenever possible before the surgical procedure in an effort to:

   a. Discover the etiology (most commonly malignancy or hyperparathyroidism)—which may in itself contribute to surgical risk—and treat the underlying disorder

   b. Treat the hypercalcemia in an effort to prevent symptoms and manifestations (discussed later), particularly adverse effects on the cardiac and neuromuscular systems

2. Clinical assessment

   a. History and physical examination

      The history and physical examination are geared toward identifying signs and symptoms that may be caused by the hypercalcemia as well as discovering the etiology.

      (1) Manifestations and symptoms

      (a) Neuromuscular: Muscle weakness, lethargy, fatigue, depressed reflexes, coma

      (b) Cardiovascular: Primary and secondary atrioventricular (AV) block owing to depressed AV nodal conduction,[1] increased ventricular irritability and automaticity, and enhancement of toxic effects of digitalis.[2] Reversible hypertension may also occur.

      (c) Gastrointestinal: Thirst, anorexia, nausea, vomiting, abdominal pain, constipation, pancreatitis, peptic ulcer disease

      (d) Renal: Nephrolithiasis, nephrocalcinosis, nephrogenic diabetes insipidus, dehydration

**TABLE 8–1. Etiologies of Hypercalcemia**

Malignancy
  Direct involvement of bone: Metastasis, leukemia, multiple
    myeloma (also osteoclast activating factor)
  No evidence of bone metastasis: Ectopic parathyroid hormone
    production
Hyperparathyroidism (and multiple endocrine neoplasia)
Hyperthyroidism
Sarcoidosis
Hyperproteinemia states (increases calcium binding)
Renal failure (acute or chronic)
Vitamin D or A toxicity
Paget's disease
Milk-alkali syndrome
Thiazine diuretics
Adrenal insufficiency
Immobilization

---

      (e) Soft-tissue calcification: May lead to band keratopathy, periarthritis, arterial calcification

    (2) Etiologies: Refer to Table 8–1 for a complete list of the etiologies of hypercalcemia. The most common in the perioperative period include:

      (a) Endocrine: One of the most frequent causes is true hyperparathyroidism, most often caused by parathyroid adenoma; less often, associated with multiple endocrine neoplasia.

      (b) Malignancy: Hypercalcemia in malignancy may occur owing to osteolytic bone metastasis, release of a parathyroidlike hormone, or release of another hormonal substance from the tumor (e.g., osteoclast activating factor; prostaglandin E).

      (c) Immobilization: Prolonged bed rest may cause or aggravate hypercalcemia. This effect may develop rapidly and continue until the patient is mobilized.

  b. Laboratory assessment

    (1) Total serum calcium is usually maintained between 8.5 and 10.5 mg/dl. Serum calcium circulates as either a protein-bound, nondiffusable moiety (45 per cent) or an ultrafilterable, ionized moiety (55 per cent). The latter has the predominant, physiologically active influence. Because

most of the bound calcium is complexed with albumin, fluctuations in the plasma protein concentration will alter the protein-bound fraction, affecting the measured serum calcium. Changes in serum albumin of 1 mg/dl will accordingly alter the serum calcium by 0.8 mg/dl.

(2) Parathyroid hormone (PTH) should be obtained in evaluating hypercalcemia. This test result will separate the etiologies into those in which PTH is elevated (primary hyperparathyroidism and malignancies producing ectopic PTH) and those in which PTH is suppressed (all others). In primary hyperparathyroidism, PTH will be inappropriately elevated for the level of calcium but may not necessarily be above "normal" range.

(3) Serum phosphorus, urinary calcium, and alkaline phosphatase provide additional diagnostic clues, as noted in Table 8–2, which reviews the more common entities.

## B. RISK ANALYSIS

1. Hypercalcemia should always be evaluated preoperatively because:
   a. The condition itself as well as its effects on the various organ systems may be exacerbated postoperatively (often owing to dehydration).
   b. The underlying etiology may adversely affect surgery.
2. Although the exact level at which hypercalcemia becomes critical in assessing surgical risk is difficult to determine, any level above 13 mg/dl should be treated promptly. Generally, levels below 11.5 mg/dl do not require immediate intervention, but the etiology should still be sought.

## C. MANAGEMENT

The most important step in treating hypercalcemia is identifying the underlying cause and tailoring therapy appropriately. However, some therapeutic interventions can be implemented to lower calcium levels rapidly.

1. Saline and furosemide

Initially, the patient should be hydrated with a normal saline solution. Six to twelve liters/day should be infused to maintain adequate urinary output (at least 3 liters/day) in the face of normal renal and cardiac function. Saline acts by volume expansion and by increasing the

**TABLE 8–2. Laboratory Assessment of Hypercalcemia**

| | PTH | Serum P | Urine CA++ | Alkaline Phosphatase |
|---|---|---|---|---|
| Hyperparathyroidism | ↑ | → | ↑ | N or ↑ |
| Metastatic carcinoma | ↓ or ↑ (ectopic PTH) | N | ↑ | N or ↑ |
| Vitamin D intoxication | → | N or ↑ | N or ↑ | N |
| Multiple myeloma | → | N | N or ↔ | N |
| Milk-alkali syndrome | → | N | N or → | N |
| Sarcoidosis | → | N or ↑ | N or ↑ | N or ↑ |
| Thyrotoxicosis | → | N | ↑ | N or ↑ |

urinary sodium and calcium excretion. It also inhibits the tubular reabsorption of calcium. If hypernatremia develops, 5% dextrose may be substituted for saline. IV furosemide (20 to 80 mg IV q4h) will help to augment a calcium diuresis. This is thought to occur owing to similar sodium and calcium handling in the kidneys. In conjunction with volume expansion, less calcium is absorbed proximally and more calcium can reach the loop of Henle, where furosemide is active, leading to its excretion. Careful attention to maintain potassium balance must be noted with the addition of 20 to 30 mEq KCl to each liter of IV fluid.

2. Glucocorticoids

Glucocorticoids may be effective therapy for hypercalcemia, especially in patients with hypervitaminosis D, sarcoidosis, tuberculosis, milk-alkali syndrome, or multiple myeloma.[3] Immobilization hypercalcemia may also be responsive to steroids.[4]

The initial dose is usually 100 to 500 mg of hydrocortisone IV followed by a maintenance dosage of 100 to 500 mg IV q8h or its oral equivalent.

3. Calcitonin

A third modality for treating hypercalcemia is the administration of calcitonin, a natural peptide produced in the C cells of the thyroid gland. It is used in the treatment of hypercalcemia of malignancy, Paget's disease and other diseases associated with bone resorption, and hyperparathyroidism. It inhibits resorption of calcium and phosphate from bone and increases their renal clearance. Skin testing with 1 I.U. (MRC) subcutaneously should precede the initial dose. Treatment may be maintained with 4 I.U. (MRC)/kg subcutaneously every 12 hours, with increase to 8 I.U. (MRC)/kg if the lower dosage is unsatisfactory after 1 or 2 days. A reaction to the skin test of more than erythema or a wheal constitutes a positive reaction and no further calcitonin should be administered. Hypocalcemic effects can be seen within a few hours.[5] An escape phenomenon may occur, causing resistance to the drug to develop. As a result, long-term treatment with calcitonin may be unsuccessful.

4. Mithramycin

Reversal of hypercalcemia (and hypercalciuria) can also be achieved with mithramycin, particularly with elevated calcium levels secondary to malignancy.[6] Mithramycin is a cytotoxic antibiotic with antiosteoclastic effects. The initial recommended dose of mithramycin is 15 to 25 μg/kg of body weight as a single IV bolus. Effects can be seen in 24 to 36 hours and last up to seven days. Doses may be repeated every three to four days as needed to maintain a normal calcium level. Care .must be taken not to cause hypocalcemia. Mithramycin can cause marrow suppression and hepatic toxicity, although these are uncommon in such small doses.

5. Phosphates

Phosphate loading is another mode of therapy for hypercalcemia after hydration and volume expansion have been accomplished.[7] Phosphate treatment should be used only in patients with elevated serum calcium levels and decreased serum phosphate levels (i.e., hyperparathyroidism), *not* in patients with renal disease or hyperphosphatemia. The IV preparation of phosphate should be used with caution, as overdosing may result in soft-tissue calcification, renal dysfunction, or shock. The mainstays of phosphate treatment are oral preparations and enemas. Available preparations include Neutra-Phos 250 mg phosphorus (2 or 3 capsules PO q.i.d.), Fleet Phospho-Soda 600 mg phosphorus/5 ml (1 tsp PO q.i.d.), and Fleet phosphate enema (100-ml retention enema b.i.d.)

6. Diphosphonates

A newer modality of treatment in patients with osteolytic metastasis or immobilization hypercalcemia is to use diphosphonates.[8] These agents inhibit bone resorption and usually show response in two days. The recommended dose of etidronate disodium is 200 mg PO b.i.d.

7. Hemodialysis

Hemodialysis and peritoneal dialysis have also been used to lower serum calcium levels, especially in patients with renal failure or when volume loading is contraindicated. Effects can be seen in several hours.

8. Prostaglandin inhibitors

Prostaglandin inhibitors like aspirin (1 gm PO t.i.d.) may be used, usually in chronic, long-term management of hypercalcemia,[9] especially in those patients with solid tumors.

Long-term management of the hypercalcemic patient obviously will depend on the underlying etiology. A low-calcium diet, avoiding immobilization, and an adequate fluid intake are all helpful modalities.

## II. HYPOCALCEMIA

### A. PREOPERATIVE EVALUATION

1. Purpose

   The hypocalcemic patient who is scheduled for surgery should be fully evaluated whenever possible before the operation in an effort to:

   a. Discover the etiology—which may in itself contribute to surgical risk—and treat the underlying disorder

   b. Treat the hypocalcemia in an effort to prevent symptoms and manifestations (discussed later), particularly adverse effects on the cardiovascular and neuromuscular systems

2. Clinical assessment

   a. History and physical examination

   The history and physical examination are geared toward identifying signs and symptoms that may be caused by the hypocalcemia as well as discovering the etiology.

   (1) Manifestations and symptoms

   (a) Neuromuscular: These are the most common manifestations, with augmented muscle contractions causing cramps, carpopedal spasm, and tetany. Classic findings include Trousseau's sign (carpal spasm precipitated by inflating a blood pressure cuff on the arm at a level to impede venous return for several minutes) and Chvostek's sign (a contraction of the eyelid muscles elicited by tapping on the facial nerve in front of the ear). Perioral paresthesia and paresthesia in the hands and feet may occur. Later clinical signs may include a change in mental status, papilledema, and seizures.

   (b) Cardiac: Prolongation of QT intevals owing to ST segment prolongation may occur, as well as depression of myocardial contractility. The effect of digitalis on the heart may be reduced.

   (c) Gastrointestinal: Symptoms are generally manifested as cramping and diarrhea.

   (2) Etiologies

   Refer to Table 8–3 for a full list of the etiologies of hypocalcemia. The most common in the perioperative period include:

   (a) Postoperative: After parathyroid (or thyroid)

**TABLE 8–3. Etiology of Hypocalcemia**

| | |
|---|---|
| Hypoalbuminemia | Intestinal malabsorption—bowel resection |
| Hypomagnesemia | |
| Hypoparathyroidism idiopathic, infiltrative irradiation, surgical | Multiple transfusions |
| | Drugs mithramycin gentamicin anticonvulsants |
| Acute pancreatitis | |
| Renal failure (acute and chronic) | Neoplasms |
| Altered vitamin D metabolism | |
| Hyperphosphatemia | Transfusion or albumin/plasma expanders |
| | Pseudohypoparathyroidism |

surgery, significant hypocalcemia may occur[10] within 24 to 48 hours. However, the calcium level will start returning to normal on the seventh to eighth postoperative day, assuming that not all the glands have been removed. The condition need be treated only if the patient is symptomatic (paresthesia, cramping, tetany).

(b) Transfusion related: After multiple rapid blood transfusions there may be a rise in the serum citrate concentration.[11] The citrate is able to bind with the ionized calcium and cause hypocalcemia. Slow infusion of 10% calcium gluconate for every 4 or 5 units of whole blood will prevent this occurrence. Similarly, large volumes of albumin or other plasma expanders may cause increased binding of calcium and thus decrease the total available ionized calcium.

(c) Renal disease: In renal disease, hypocalcemia is thought to be secondary to skeletal resistance to effects of PTH, failure to hydroxylate vitamin D level in the kidneys, and an elevated phosphate level.[12] However, owing to concurrent metabolic acidosis, renal failure patients have fewer episodes of symptomatic hypocalcemia.

(d) Hypoalbuminemia: Most commonly seen in sick or malnourished patients, particularly those with liver or kidney disease. Remember: for each 1 gram decrease in serum albumin, a 0.8 mg decrease in the serum calcium level occurs; because the level of ionized calcium is normal, no treatment is required.

(e) Magnesium deficiency: Seen in the severely malnourished patient or alcoholic, magnesium deficiency of a severe degree may produce profound hypocalcemia. It is felt that this develops secondary to impaired release of PTH and diminished skeletal responsiveness to PTH.[13]

b. Laboratory assessment

A total serum calcium is usually maintained between 8.5 and 10.5 mg/dl. As mentioned earlier, serum calcium level must be interpreted in combination with albumin level. Additional blood studies for evaluation of hypocalcemia include phosphate, magnesium, PTH, and vitamin D levels.

## B. RISK ANALYSIS

1. Hypocalcemia should always be evaluated preoperatively and postoperatively (in high-risk patients who are postparathyroidectomy or postthyroidectomy) because:
   a. Severe adverse effects on various organ systems may result
   b. The underlying etiology may increase the surgical risk
2. Although the exact level at which hypocalcemia becomes critical in assessing surgical risk is difficult to determine, subnormal levels should be carefully monitored, evaluated, and treated.

## C. TREATMENT

Effective management of the hypocalcemic patient involves careful monitoring of the serum calcium and phosphate levels for seven days after beginning therapy. Thereafter, less frequent determinations are made until a steady state has developed. If therapy is required for longer than three months after parathyroid surgery, permanent hypoparathyroidism is most likely and treatment should be adjusted to maintain the calcium within normal range. For details of calcium replacement, see Tables 8–4 and 8–5.

1. Intravenous calcium therapy

Calcium replacement is considered a medical emergency procedure if there is neuromuscular irritability or

TABLE 8–4. Calcium Preparations—Oral

| Type | Tablet | Mg of Calcium |
|------|--------|---------------|
| Calcium gluconate | 500 mg | 45 |
| Calcium lactate | 325 mg | 42.25 |
| Calcium carbonate | 650 mg | 260 |
| (OS-Cal 500) | 1.25 gm | 500 |
| Calcium glubionate (syrup) | 1.8 gm/5 ml | 115 |

CNS manifestations. An initial infusion of 10 to 20 ml of 10% calcium gluconate should be given over 15 minutes. This can be followed with a titrated infusion drip to maintain a calcium level of 8 to 8.5 mg/dl. In the patient who is predisposed to hypomagnesemia (alcohol, malabsorption, parenteral feedings) a single dose of 1 gm of magnesium sulfate IM or IV is recommended once a serum magnesium level is sent. Pending this result, repeat dosing every four to six hours may be necessary. Once the patient is stable, the underlying cause of hypocalcemia should be identified and treated accordingly.

2. Oral calcium therapy

If chronic replacement is necessary, a patient should be started on an oral calcium preparation. The recommended daily maintenance of calcium is 800 to 1000 mg/day for the average adult. However, in calcium-depleted patients, 1 to 2 gm/day is usually administered in three or four divided doses.

TABLE 8–5. Calcium Preparations—Intravenous*

| Type of Calcium | % Solution | Mg Elemental Ca$^+$ | μg Ca$^+$/gm or 10 ml† |
|-----------------|-----------|---------------------|------------------------|
| Calcium chloride‡ | 10 | 272 | 13.6 |
| Calcium gluconate§ | 10 | 90 | 4.5 |
| Calcium gluceptate | 22 | 90 | 4.5 |
| Calcium levulinate | 10 | 130 | 6.9 |

*Caution not to mix calcium solutions with $HCO_3^-$ because of tendency to precipitate calcium salts
†Often available on emergency carts in 10-ml vials
‡May be extremely irritating to tissues if extravasated
§Preferred IM preparation

## REFERENCES

1. Watanabe Y: Effects of Ca Ha concentrations on A-V conduction: Experimental study in rabbit hearts with clinical implications on heart block and slow calcium channel blocking agents. Am Heart J 102:883, 1981.
2. Ream A, Fugdall R: Acute Cardiovascular Management. Philadelphia, JB Lippincott, 1982.
3. Carroll HJ, Oh MS: Water, Electrolyte, and Acid–Base Metabolism. Philadelphia, JB Lippincott, 1978.
4. Henke JA et al: Immobilization hypercalcemic crisis. Arch Surg 110:321, 1975.
5. Deftos L: Calcitonin as a drug. Ann Intern Med 95:192–197, 1981.
6. Edwards CRW, Besser GM: Mitramycin treatment of malignant hypercalcemia. Br Med J 3:167, 1968.
7. Massry SG: Inorganic phosphate treatment of hypercalcemia. Arch Intern Med 121:307, 1968.
8. Merli GJ, et al: Immobilization hypercalcemia in acute spinal cord injury treated with disodium etidronate. Arch Intern Med 144:1286, 1984.
9. Syberth HW, et al: Prostaglandins as mediators of hypercalcemia with cancer. N Engl J Med 293:1278, 1975.
10. Jones KH, Fourman P: Prevalence of parathyroid insufficiency after thyroidectomy. Lancet 2:721, 1963.
11. Clowes GHA, Simeone FA: Acute hypocalcemia in surgical patients. Ann Surg 146:539, 1957.
12. Morrison G, Murray TG: Electrolyte, acid–base, and fluid homeostasis in chronic renal failure. Med Clin North Am 65:429, 1981.
13. Reddy CR, et al: Studies on the mechanism of hypocalcemia of magnesium depletion. J Clin Invest 52:3000, 1973.

# 9

## PHEOCHROMOCYTOMA

## I. PREOPERATIVE EVALUATION

### A. PURPOSE

The pheochromocytoma is a catecholamine-secreting tumor. An estimated 10,000 to 20,000 patients have this curable form of hypertension—but these are from a pool of 20 million hypertensives.[1] The possibility of pheochromocytoma is important to consider for the following reasons:

1. The tumor always enters a differential diagnosis of hypertension.
2. Surgical mortality with appropriate medical treatment is low.[2]
3. If the tumor goes unrecognized, associated surgery may have a high mortality.[3]

### B. CLINICAL ASSESSMENT

1. History and physical examination

   Clinical findings include hypertension (either in paroxysms or sustained) and symptoms of adrenergic excess. Most common symptoms include headache, diaphoresis, palpitations, tachycardia, pallor, anxiety and nervousness, tremor, nausea, anorexia, fatigue, weight loss, and postural hypotension.

   Similar symptoms may result from other etiologies, which must be considered in the differential diagnosis of pheochromocytoma. These include thyrotoxicosis, hypoglycemia, anxiety, coronary artery insufficiency, brain tumor, carcinoid syndrome, hypertensive crises of other etiologies, menopause, and drugs.

2. Laboratory assessment

   a. Urinary vanillylmandelic acid (VMA) and metanephrine determinations are sufficient biochemical testing for most cases of pheochromocytoma. However, plasma catecholamines has been advocated as the test of choice by some.[4]

b. Vanillylmandelic acid and metanephrines should be measured and reported as micrograms per milligram creatinine. This eliminates collection errors. Determination of total metanephrines has produced the fewest false-negative results. Many screening tests for pheochromocytoma are used. These tests are notoriously nonspecific and give many false-positive results because they test merely for phenolic acids, which are present in many drugs, foods, and drinks—including raw fruit, vanilla, and coffee. Routine tests must be confirmed by more specific tests, such as high-pressure liquid chromatography. These results have been highly specific and sensitive.[5] Normal values for each study should be obtained from the specific laboratory that is used.

c. In general, a number of clinical states and drugs can interfere with biochemical determinants (see Tables 9–1 and 9–2). Drugs that lack sufficient effect to alter diagnostic results with quantitative VMA on metanephrine determination are listed in Table 9–3.

d. Once the diagnosis is strongly suggested by clinical and biochemical studies, the tumor should be localized. In adults, 90 per cent are found in the adrenal; 10 per cent are extra-adrenal. Ten per cent are bilateral. Computerized tomography is the best method of preoperative localization. If the adrenal glands are negative, scans including the remainder of the abdomen and pelvis should be done. If scanning is unsuccessful, selective venous sampling may help approximate the tumor's location.

## II. MANAGEMENT

### A. PREOPERATIVE

Adequate alpha adrenergic blockade with oral phenoxybenzamine should be established before invasive procedures or surgery. The dose is begun at 10 mg twice daily and increased until blood pressure is adequately controlled.

**TABLE 9–1. Conditions That Increase VMA and Metanephrine Excretion Without Pheochromocytoma**

Head trauma
Coma or increased intracranial pressure
Hemorrhagic shock
Severe stress

**TABLE 9–2. Drugs That May Alter Detection of Urinary VMA or Metanephrines Significantly**

**Metanephrines**

Increase: Chlorpromazine, monoamine oxidase inhibitors, levodopa, methocarbamol, trihexyphenidyl

Decrease: X-ray contrast media containing methylglucamine (Renografin, Renovist, Hypaque)

**VMA**

Increase: Nalidixic acid, levodopa, methocarbamol, trihexyphenidyl

Decrease: Monoamine oxidase inhibitors, clofibrate

Average dose is 40 to 120 mg/day, but doses as high as 200 mg/day may be needed. Side effects include nasal congestion, xerostomia, sedation, and orthostatic hypotension. One to two weeks of preoperative treatment generally are recommended. Beta blockade is not essential but should be used to treat significant tachycardia or arrhythmias. Beta blockers should never be given before establishment of adequate alpha blockade, since severe hypertension could occur owing to unopposed alpha vasoconstriction.

## B. INTRAOPERATIVE

Phentolamine (a short-acting alpha blocker) or nitroprusside should be available during surgery or invasive diagnostic procedures. Nitroprusside is preferred, since blood pressure can be more easily controlled owing to its continuous infusion with rapid onset and brief duration of action. Arterial line monitoring should accompany this therapy. Infusion can be discontinued immediately on clamping the adrenal vein, limiting the rapid drop in blood pressure during

**TABLE 9–3. Drugs with Insufficient Effect to Alter Diagnostic Results with Quantitative VMA or Metanephrine Determination**

| | |
|---|---|
| Diuretics | Digitalis |
| Methyldopa (except for high dose) | Meprobamate |
| Reserpine | Spironolactone |
| Guanethidine | Epinephrine |
| Most antihistamines | Dextroamphetamine |
| Acetylsalicylic acid | Chlorothiazide |
| Phenobarbital | Phenylephrine |
| | Isoproterenol |

TABLE 9–4. Intraoperative Dosages for Pheochromocytoma Surgery

| Hypertensive Episodes | |
|---|---|
| Nitroprusside | 0.5–1 µg/kg/min initially to maximum of 10 µg/kg/min |
| Phentolamine | 1–5 mg IV at 1 mg/min |
| **Arrhythmias** | |
| Propranolol | 1 mg/minute IV up to 5 mg |
| Lidocaine | 50 to 100 mg IV bolus followed by 1–4 mg/min infusion |

tumor removal. Phentolamine can be given only in IV bolus and thus titration of blood pressure is difficult. Arrhythmias may be controlled with propranolol or lidocaine. See Table 9–4 for drug dosages.

## III. POSTOPERATIVE

Severe hypotension may follow tumor removal as a result of volume depletion or adrenergic unresponsiveness. Volume replacement with plasma or albumin in saline usually is corrective. Vasoconstrictors are rarely needed.

Postoperative hypertension may be caused by overhydration, renal disease, accidental renal artery ligation, persistent tumor, essential hypertension, or continued release of stored catecholamines. Such hypertension is best treated with conventional therapy in the presence of a confident surgical report. Postoperative urine collection of catecholamines should be delayed for several weeks owing to the possibility of continued release from stores in sympathetic nerve endings.

Steroid replacement will be necessary if both adrenal glands are removed.

Postoperative hypoglycemia has also been reported, and glucose levels should be followed.

## REFERENCES

1. Fernandes M. Bellini G: Management of the patient with pheochromocytoma. Drug Therapy, May 1977, p 43.

2. DeOreo GA, Steward BH, Tarazi RC, Gifford RW: Preoperative blood transfusion in safe surgical management of pheochromocytoma: A review of 46 cases. J Urol *3*:715, 1974.

3. Apgor V, Papper FM: Pheochromocytoma—anesthetic management during surgical treatment. Arch Surg *62*:634, 1951.

4. Bravo EL, et al: Circulatory and urinary catecholamines in pheochromocytoma. N Engl J Med *301*:682, 1979.

5. Sheps SG, VanHeerden JA, Sheedy PF: Uncontrollable hypertension: Is it pheochromocytoma? Consultant, November 1980, p 153.

Preoperative evaluation and management of patients with gastrointestinal disease is complicated by the large number of potential risk factors, which depend on the specific disease entity. Two common links that are of concern in all patients with gastrointestinal disease are possible nutritional debilitation and postoperative disorders in pulmonary function after abdominal surgery. Specific problems that may arise during the perioperative period related to gastrointestinal disease are discussed later.

## I. DIVERTICULITIS

### A. PREOPERATIVE EVALUATION

1. Background and purpose

   Diverticulitis occurs in about 20 per cent to 25 per cent of patients with diverticulosis.[1, 2, 3] The cause of diverticulitis is probably mechanical, related to retention in the diverticula of undigested food residues and bacteria. This compromises the blood supply to the thin-walled sac and renders it susceptible to invasion by colonic bacteria. Complications, such as perforation, abscess, fistula, obstruction, and hemorrhage, occur in 20 per cent of patients with acute diverticulitis.[4] The aim of the internist is to treat the patient during the initial episode and to prepare the patient for surgery if it becomes necessary.

2. Clinical assessment

   a. Complications:[5] The concern of the internist is to assess the patient's medical status and determine if complications of diverticular disease exist. Figure 10–1 illustrates the complications that occur in 20 per cent of patients with acute diverticulitis.

   (1) Hemorrhage: Massive hemorrhage with melena may occur in 5 per cent to 27 per cent of patients

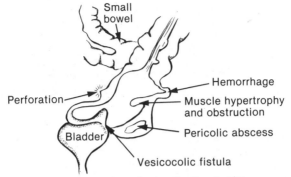

**Figure 10–1.** Complications in diverticulitis.

with noninflamed diverticular disease.[2] Occult bleeding is by far a more common manifestation of diverticular disease.

(2) Obstruction: An average of 20 per cent of patients undergoing surgery for diverticulitis have obstruction. Obstruction is more commonly incomplete.[6]

(3) Perforation: Although microperforation usually occurs with acute diverticulitis, rupture of a diverticulum with generalized fecal peritonitis is relatively uncommon (2 per cent to 4 per cent of patients).[1,2]

(4) Abscess: Abscess has been noted in between 10 per cent and 28 per cent of surgical cases. Generally, the symptoms of diverticulitis do not subside in three to five days, and progressive abdominal symptoms increase, with some patients developing a palpable left lower quadrant mass.[1,2,7]

(5) Fistula: Colovesical fistulas are present in 6 per cent to 23 per cent of patients undergoing surgery for diverticulitis and occur five times more often in men than in women.[1,2,7] Coloenteric, colocolonic, and colovaginal fistulas are uncommon. Colocutaneous fistulas are nearly always the result of surgical drainage of a pericolic abscess.

(6) Recurrence:[4] Recurrent episodes of diverticulitis are seen in 45 per cent of patients. The incidence of recurrence after surgery is low, with 57 per

cent to 89 per cent of patients remaining symptom-free.[8, 9, 10, 11, 12]

  b. Laboratory studies

    (1) CBC with platelets

    (2) Electrolytes, BUN, and glucose

    (3) Prothrombin time and partial thromboplastin time

    (4) Urinalysis

    (5) ECG

    (6) Chest x-ray

    (7) Abdominal x-ray series, flat plate and upright

## B. PERIOPERATIVE MANAGEMENT

1. Prophylaxis: This regimen should be followed in *all* patients undergoing elective surgery.[13]

  a. Neomycin 1 gm and erythromycin 1 gm PO at 1:00 P.M., 2:00 P.M., and 11:00 P.M. the day before surgery.

  b. For patients who are unable to take medication by mouth, give doxycycline 200 mg IV, or cefoxitin 1 gm IV at the induction of anesthesia.

2. Prophylaxis for endocarditis: see Chapter 2.

3. Therapeutic regimen: For patients with fever or leukocytosis, or for those undergoing emergency surgery, give:

  a. Aminoglycoside    1.5 mg/kg loading; then 1 mg/kg q8h IV

    plus

    clindamycin      600 mg q8h IV

    *or*

  b. Cefoxitin        1 gm q4–8h IV

## II. GASTRIC AND PEPTIC ULCER DISEASE

## A. PREOPERATIVE EVALUATION

1. Background and purpose

    The term peptic ulcer refers to the major group of duodenal and gastric ulcers in which acid pepsin appears to have played a pathogenetic role. Duodenal ulcers are estimated to occur in 10 per cent of the population between the third and fourth decades.[14] Gastric ulcers have their peak incidence in the sixth decade.[14] In the preoperative evaluation of this patient population, the age, concomitant disease, type of ulcer complication, and surgical procedure must be considered in the estimation of surgical risk.

**TABLE 10–1. Age-Related Mortality**

| Study | Age | No. of Patients | No. of Deaths | % | Total in Study |
|-------|-----|-----------------|---------------|---|----------------|
| Irvin & Zeppa[15] | 80 | 10 | 9 | 90% | 347 |
| Pillay et al.[16] | 75 | 37 | 8 | 21.6% | 37 |

2. Clinical assessment

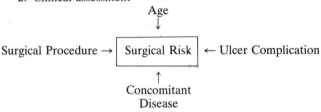

a. Age: In two studies listed in Table 10–1, the increased incidence of mortality is demonstrated with respect to age.
b. Complications:[14] First to be considered in this group of patients is the incidence of hemorrhage, perforation, and obstruction. Hemorrhage occurs in approximately 15 per cent to 20 per cent and recurrence of bleeding, in about 40 per cent. Perforation into the peritoneal cavity presents in 6 per cent of patients, and in 10 per cent of these there is concomitant hemorrhage. Obstruction occurs in only 2 per cent to 4 per cent of patients, and symptoms usually have been present for a long time. The second consideration is whether the surgical procedure was elective or emergent. Tables 10–2 and 10–3 list the mortality with respect to each of these two factors.
c. Concomitant disease: In Irvin and Zeppa's study,[15] four preoperative disease groups were assessed, and renal disease was weighted the highest. Table 10–4 lists the mortality related to each.
d. Surgical procedure: Irvin and Zeppa[15] and Wolf and associates[17] both state that vagotomy and antrectomy, or vagotomy and pyloroplasty, have the same mortality and did not influence operative risk. The former affords the best procedure to prevent reulceration.[15, 16]

**TABLE 10–2. Ulcer Complications and Mortality**

| Study | Complication | Total Pts. | Deaths | Mortality (%) |
|-------|-------------|------------|--------|---------------|
| Irvin & Zeppa[15] | Hemorrhage | 157 | 22 | 14 |
| | Perforation | 77 | 13 | 17 |
| | Obstruction | 57 | 1 | 2 |
| | | | | |
| *Pillay et al.[16] | Hemorrhage | 20 | 5 | 25 |
| | Perforation | 13 | 3 | 23 |
| | Obstruction | 1 | 0 | 0 |
| | | | | |
| *Wolf et al.[17] | Hemorrhage | 44 | 12 | 27.2 |
| | Perforation | 32 | 3 | 9 |
| | Obstruction | 0 | 0 | 0 |

*Emergency surgery.

**TABLE 10–3. Emergency Ulcer Surgery and Mortality**

| Study | Emergency Surgery | Deaths | Mortality (%) |
|-------|-------------------|--------|---------------|
| Irvin & Zeppa[15] | 126 | 32 | 25.3 |
| Pillay et al.[16] | 37 | 8 | 21.6 |
| Wolf et al.[17] | 76 | 15 | 19.7 |

**TABLE 10–4. Mortality and Preoperative Disease**

| Disease Group | Total | Survivors | Deaths |
|---------------|-------|-----------|--------|
| Pulmonary | 24 | 18 | 6 (25%) |
| Cardiovascular | 18 | 15 | 3 (17%) |
| Renal | 13 | 9 | 4 (31%) |
| Hepatic | 7 | 5 | 2 (29%) |
| Total | 62 | 47 | 15 (24%) |

e. Laboratory studies
   (1) CBC with platelets
   (2) Electrolytes, BUN, glucose
   (3) Creatinine
   (4) Liver function
   (5) Type and cross-match
   (6) ECG
   (7) Chest x-ray
   (8) Obstruction series

## B. PERIOPERATIVE MANAGEMENT

1. Fluid therapy: Appropriate fluids should be administered to maintain blood volume.
2. Antibiotics
   a. Prophylaxis: Cefazolin 1 gr IM on call to the operating room, or IV with the induction of anesthesia
   b. Prophylaxis for endocarditis: See Chapter 2.

# III. CHOLECYSTECTOMY

## A. PREOPERATIVE EVALUATION

1. Background and purpose
   Acute cholecystitis occurs in more than 90 per cent of patients with obstruction of the cystic duct by calculi, and in 50 per cent of patients with cholelithiasis. The aim of preoperative evaluation is to assess the risk of surgical removal of the gallbladder and to determine the need for antibiotic coverage. With respect to antibiotic usage, the approach can be one of prophylaxis or of prescribing a therapeutic regimen for patients with biliary tract disease.
2. Clinical assessment
   a. Pulmonary: This is a critical area to assess, since the vital capacity falls to 25 per cent of the preoperative value with upper abdominal surgery (Fig. 10–2).[18]
   b. Laboratory studies
      (1) CBC with platelets
      (2) Electrolytes, BUN, glucose
      (3) Creatinine
      (4) Liver function
      (5) Bilirubin (total and direct)
      (6) Prothrombin time and partial thromboplastin time
      (7) Pulmonary function
      (8) Urinalysis
      (9) Chest x-ray and flat plate of abdomen

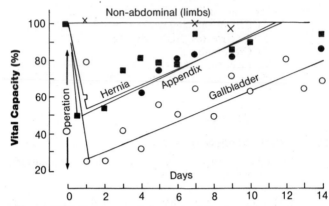

**Figure 10–2.** Pulmonary vital capacity following abdominal surgery. (Adapted from Churchill, E.D., and McNeil, D.: Surg. Gynecol. Obstet., 44:483–488, 1927.)

(10) ECG
(11) Ultrasound of gallbladder

## B. PERIOPERATIVE MANAGEMENT

1. Prophylaxis: The following patients undergoing elective surgery should receive prophylaxis,[19] as indicated:

   a. Over age 70 ⎫ Cefazolin 1 gm IM on call to
   b. Previous biliary tract ⎪ the operating room or IV with
      surgery ⎪ induction of anesthesia
   c. Obstructive jaundice ⎬
   d. Common bile duct ⎪
      obstruction without ⎪
      jaundice ⎭

2. Prophylaxis for endocarditis: See Chapter 2.

3. Therapeutic regimen: These patients have fever and leukocytosis secondary to acute cholecystitis, cholangitis, or septicemia from biliary tract disease, and antibiotics are definitely indicated. Observe one of the following regimens:

   a. Aminoglycoside 1.5 mg/kg q8h *plus* ampicillin 1 gm q6h

   b. Aminoglycoside 1.5 mg/kg q8h *plus* cefoxitin 2 gm q6–8h *or* cefamandole 1 gm q4–6h

   c. If patient is allergic to penicillin, aminoglycoside 1.5 mg/kg q8h *plus* chloramphenicol 50 mg/kg/day at six-hour intervals

4. Prophylaxis for deep vein thrombosis (DVT) and pulmonary embolism (PE): Patients with risk factors should receive the prophylaxis indicated:

a. Over age 40           ⎤ Heparin 5000 U subcuta-
b. Obesity                  │ neously two hours before
c. Varicose veins          │ surgery, then 5000 U sub-
d. Previous DVT and PE   │ cutaneously 8 to 12 hours
e. Malignancy             │ after the initial dose until
f. Immobilization        ⎦ the patient is discharged

5. Pulmonary: Since there is a reduction in vital capacity, good postural drainage, percussion, and deep breathing should be encouraged postoperatively by the nursing staff or the respiratory therapist.

## C. SPECIAL CONSIDERATION

1. Organisms
   The choice of antibiotic will be influenced by the flora noted in the bile of patients with biliary tract disease. Table 10–5 shows the most common flora seen in biliary disease in the 231 patients studied by Keighley and coworkers.[20]

2. Antibiotics
   The bile concentration of antibiotics is not obtainable in acute cholecystitis; thus adequate serum and tissue concentrations are the important goals to achieve with the regimen.[21]

**TABLE 10–5. Common Bacteria in Biliary Disease**

| | | |
|---|---|---|
| *Escherichia coli* | 65 | (36) |
| *Klebsiella aerogenes, Aerobacter* spp. | 20 | (12) |
| *Streptococcus baccalis* | 22 | (15) |
| *Proteus* spp. | 13 | (12) |
| *Enterobacter cloacae* | 8 | (6) |
| *Streptococcus viridens* | 3 | (1) |
| *Pseudomonas aeruginosa* | 3 | (2) |
| *Serratia* spp. | 2 | (0) |
| *Aeromonas* spp. | 1 | (0) |
| *Lactobacillus* spp. | 1 | (0) |
| *Staphylococcus aureus* | 2 | (1) |
| *Staphylococcus albus* | 3 | (2) |
| *Paracolon* spp. | 1 | (1) |
| Others | 2 | |
| Anaerobic streptococci | 7 | (3) |
| *Clostridium* | 11 | (1) |
| *Bacteroides* spp. | 2 | (2) |
| Total | 106 | (104) |

## IV. ACUTE PANCREATITIS

### A. PREOPERATIVE EVALUATION

1. Background and purpose
   The incidence of pancreatitis varies depending on the etiologic factors. In the United States, alcohol is the most common cause, with cholelithiasis the second most frequently recognized etiology.[22] The initial challenge is establishing the correct diagnosis, since medical versus surgical management could alter the patient's prognosis. Second, the degree of pancreatitis must be assessed, using the history, physical examination, and laboratory data. The consultant should combine these two aspects to provide a better assessment of preoperative risk.

2. Clinical assessment
   a. Figure 10–3 shows the three most common causes of pancreatitis and three reasons for surgery.
   b. Objective signs to estimate the severity of pancreatitis associated with various etiologies are shown in Table 10–6.[23]
   c. Timing of surgery
      (1) Early: Patients with mild pancreatitis have an associated 7.7 per cent mortality. Patients with severe pancreatitis have a 44 per cent mortality.
      (2) Late: Patients with previous episodes of pancreatitis secondary to cholethiasis have a risk of subsequent pancreatitis of between 36 per cent and 63 per cent. Surgery in this group has been reported as carrying little risk.[24, 25]

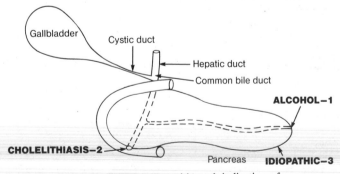

**Figure 10–3.** Causes of pancreatitis and indications for surgery. Reasons to operate: (a) Deterioration in clinical state; (b) jaundice; (c) acute abdomen of unknown etiology.

**TABLE 10–6. Evaluation of Pancreatitis**

| At Admission or Diagnosis | During Initial 48 Hours |
|---|---|
| Over age 55 y | Hct < 10% |
| WBC > 16,000/cu mm | BUN < 5 mg/100 ml |
| Glucose > 200 mg/100 ml | Serum $Ca^{++}$ < 8 mg/100 ml |
| LDH > 350 IU/liter | Base deficit < 4 mEq/liter |
| SGOT > units/100 ml | Fluid sequestration > 6000 ml |
| | $Po_2$ < 60 mm Hg |

    d. Laboratory studies
       (1) CBC with platelets
       (2) Electrolytes, BUN, glucose
       (3) Prothrombin time and partial thromboplastin time
       (4) Serum amylase and clearance
       (5) Serum calcium and albumin
       (6) Serum magnesium in the alcoholic
       (7) Liver enzymes
       (8) Arterial blood gas
       (9) Chest x-ray
      (10) ECG
      (11) Abdominal x-ray series (KUB and upright abdomen)

## B. PERIOPERATIVE MANAGEMENT

  1. Analgesia: Meperidine 50 to 100 mg IM plus hydroxyzine 50 to 100 mg q4h as needed for pain.
  2. Diet: The patient is kept NPO, with nasogastric suction.
  3. Thiamine 100 mg IM once a day in the alcoholic patient.
  4. Fluid therapy: Maintain adequate fluid balance and replace appropriate electrolytes to include calcium and magnesium.
  5. Antibiotics
    a. Prophylaxis:[26] If an exploratory laparotomy is performed to rule out a mechanical cause of obstruction, prophylactic antibiotics should be used in the following patient population:
      (1) Over age 70
      (2) Previous biliary tract surgery
      (3) Obstructive jaundice

    Cefazolin 1 gm IM on call to the operating room or IV with induction of anesthesia

        (4) Common duct
           obstruction
           without jaundice

  b. Prophylaxis for endocarditis: See Chapter 2.

  c. Therapeutic regimen: If, associated with the pancreatitis, the patient has fever and leukocytosis, full antibiotic therapy must be used.

      (1) Aminoglycoside 1.5 mg/kg q8h *plus* ampicillin 1 gm q6h

      (2) Aminoglycoside 1.5 mg/kg q8h *plus* cefoxitin 2 gm q6–8h *or* cefamandazole 1 gm q4–6h

      (3) If patient is allergic to penicillin, aminoglycoside 1.5 mg/kg q8h *plus* chloramphenicol 50 mg/kg/day at six-hour intervals

## REFERENCES

### Diverticulitis

1. Parks TG: Natural history of diverticular disease of the colon. A review of 521 cases. Br Med J *4*:639, 1969.
2. Berman PM, Kirner JB: Current knowledge of diverticular disease of the colon. Am J Dig Dis *17*:741, 1972.
3. Boles RS, Jr, Jordan SM: The clinical significance of diverticulosis. Gastroenterology *35*:579, 1958.
4. Roth LA: Complications of colonic diverticulitis. Postgrad Med *60*:115–118, 1976.
5. Barbezat GO: Rational treatment of diverticular disease. Drugs *19*:63–69, 1980.
6. Botsford TW, Zollinger RM Jr: Diverticulitis of the colon. Surg Gynecol Obstet *128*:1209, 1969.
7. Hughes LE: Complications of diverticular disease. Clin Gastroenterol *4*:147–170, 1975.
8. Moseley RV, Ross FP: Sigmoid diverticulitis: Evaluation of current practice in a community hospital. Ann Surg *164*:275–283, 1966.
9. Leigh JE, Judd ES, Waugh JM: Diverticulitis of the colon after apparently adequate segmental resection. Am J Surg *103*:51–54, 1962.
10. Bolt BE, Hughes LE: Diverticulitis: A follow-up of 100 cases. Br Med J *1*:1205–1209, 1966.
11. Levy SB, Fit WT, Lench JB: Surgical treatment of diverticular disease of the colon: Evaluation of an eleven-year period. Ann Surg *166*:947–954, 1967.
12. Wychules AR, Beahrs OH, Judd ES: Surgical management of diverticulitis of the colon. Surg Clin North Am *47*:961–969, 1967.
13. Antimicrobial prophylaxis for surgery. The Medical Letter *23*:77, 1981.

*Gastric and Peptic Ulcer Disease*

14. McGuigan JE: Peptic ulcer, in Thorn GW, et al (eds): Principles of Internal Medicine, McGraw-Hill, 9th ed. New York, 1980, Ch 290.
15. Irvin G, Zeppa R: Predicted survival in peptic ulcer patients based on computer analysis of preoperative variables. Ann Surg
16. Pillay S, Hardie I, Burnett W: Emergency surgery for complications of peptic ulcer in the elderly. Aust NZJ Surg *51*:590, 1981.
17. Wolf J, Bell C, Zimberg Y: Analysis of 10 years' experience with surgery for peptic ulcer disease. Am Surg, April 1972, p 187.

*Cholecystectomy*

18. Churchill ED, McNeil D: The reduction in vital capacity following operation. Surg Gynecol Obstet *44*:483–488, 1927.
19. Hirschmann JV: Rational antibiotic prophylaxis. Hosp Pract, November 1981, p 105.
20. Keighley MEB, et al: Antibiotic treatment of biliary sepsis. Surg Clin North Am *55*:1379, 1975.
21. Jarvinen B, Renkonen O, Palmu A: Antibiotics in acute cholecystitis. Ann Clin Res *10*:247, 1978.

*Acute Pancreatitis*

22. Greenberger N, Toskes P, Isselbacher K: Disease of the Pancreas, in Thorn GW, et al (eds): Harrison's Principles of Internal Medicine, 9th ed. New York, McGraw-Hill, 1980, Ch 309.
23. Ranson JH, et al: Prognostic signs and the role of operative management in acute pancreatitis. Surg Gynecol Obstet *139*:69, 1974.
24. Ranson JH: The timing of biliary surgery in acute pancreatitis. Ann Surg *189*:654, 1979.
25. Paloyan D, Skinner DB: The timing of biliary tract operations in patients with pancreatitis associated with gallstones. Surg Gynecol Obstet *141*:737, 1975.
26. Hirschmann JV: Rational antibiotic prophylaxic. Hosp Pract, November 1981, p 105.

# LIVER DISEASE

Surgery in patients with liver disease must be approached with an understanding of the physiologic effect of anesthesia and extra-anesthetic factors on the splanchnic circulation. Such anesthetic agents as cyclopropane, halothane, methoxyflurane, and nitrous oxide all reduce spanchnic blood flow by various mechanisms. Cyclopropane activates the sympathetic nervous system, which results in splanchnic vasoconstriction.[1] Halothane and methoxyflurane diminish cardiac output, which decreases perfusion through the splanchnic bed.[1] Nitrous oxide hyperventilation anesthesia results in diminished flow and overventilation, which leads to increased splanchnic vascular resistance and decreased flow.[1] The extraanesthetic factors, such as visceral traction, blood loss, positive airway pressure, and changes in $P_{CO_2}$, alter splanchnic blood flow, either through sympathetic activity or through reflex mechanism—all of which decrease liver flow.[2]

The following sections review acute parenchymal, cholestatic, and chronic parenchymal liver disease. The physiologic effects of anesthesia and extraanesthetic factors are correlated with the respective liver disease process so that risk can be determined with some accuracy.

## V. VIRAL HEPATITIS

### A. PREOPERATIVE EVALUATION

1. Background and purpose

    The most common cause of hepatitis is infection with viral agents type A, type B, and non-A, non-B. Other causes of infectious hepatitis are coxsackievirus, Epstein-Barr virus, cytomegalovirus, and herpes simplex virus type 2.

    Table 10–7 shows the clinical and epidemiologic difference between the various types of viral hepatitis. Hepatitis A, formerly infectious hepatitis, is the etiologic agent in 25 per cent of sporadic cases of hepatitis.[3] The incubation period is short, and the virus is communicated by the oral–fecal route. Hepatitis B, or serum hepatitis, accounts for 50 per cent of the sporadic cases. The incubation period is long, and it is spread by the parenteral route. Of patients with acute hepatitis B 10 per cent to 20 per cent become carriers. Hepatitis non-A, non-B has a short (2 wk) and a long (6 mo) incubation period. This agent accounts for the other 25 per cent of sporadic cases of hepatitis but is the cause in 90 per cent of post-transfusional hepatitis. The mode of transmission is parenteral. Chronic hepatitis develops in 10 per cent to 20 per cent of sporadic cases and in 40 per cent to 60 per cent of post-transfusion cases.[4]

    Having reviewed the background of these three hepatic infections, preoperative evaluation is aimed at assessing the degree of hepatic compromise and its concomitant problems. The consultant must always recall that anesthesia decreases hepatic blood flow and could further exacerbate hepatic disease.

**TABLE 10–7. Seroepidemiologic Characteristics of Viral Hepatitis***

| Type | Incubation | Mode of Spread | Contagious Body Fluids | Diagnostic Serology | Carrier State | Severe Chronic Liver Disease |
|---|---|---|---|---|---|---|
| Hepatitis A | 2–6 weeks | Fecal-oral, sporadic, epidemic Contaminated food or water | Stool | Acute: IgM anti-HA Delayed: IgG anti-HA | Negative | Negative |
| Hepatitis B | 6 weeks–6 months | Close contact (parenteral, sexual) | Blood, saliva, semen | Acute: HB$_s$Ag, anti-HB$_c$ Delayed: anti-HB$_s$ | Positive (10%) | Positive (2%–3%) |
| Non-A, non-B hepatitis | 2 weeks–6 months (short and long) | Parenteral, sporadic | Blood(?) | | Positive | Positive (2%–20%) |

*From Medical Knowledge Self-Assessment Program VI, Chapter on Gastroenterology, American College of Physicians, 1982, p. 74.

2. Clinical assessment
   a. Fulminant hepatitis will develop in 1 per cent to 2 per cent of patients with viral hepatitis and carries a 75 per cent mortality.[5] Hepatitis B is the most common cause of fulminant hepatitis.
   b. Signs of active hepatitis (jaundice, hepatomegaly) should be determined.
   c. Laboratory studies
      (1) CBC with platelets
      (2) Electrolytes, BUN, and glucose
      (3) Prothrombin time and partial thromboplastin time
      (4) SGOT, SGPT, alkaline phosphatase, bilirubin, albumin
      (5) Creatinine
      (6) Urinalysis
      (7) Chest x-ray
      (8) ECG
      (9) Hepatitis serology

## B. PERIOPERATIVE MANAGEMENT AND RISK

1. Appropriate precautions and prophylaxis must be followed pre- and postoperatively in a patient with hepatitis.
2. Surgery in patients with viral hepatitis has been associated with an increased mortality as high as 9.5 per cent.[6] Therefore, if possible, delay of surgery is the best approach until one month after the liver enzymes return to normal.

## VI. ALCOHOLIC LIVER DISEASE

## A. PREOPERATIVE EVALUATION

1. Background and purpose
   Alcoholic liver disease is one of the most common causes of hepatic dysfunction, occurring in 10 per cent to 20 per cent of a population of heavy drinkers. In the United States, this is estimated to be about 15 to 20 million persons. The extent of hepatic damage depends on the quantity of alcohol consumed, the length of time the patient has been drinking, and the patient's general nutritional status and most likely is modified by genetic predisposition. Acute hepatocellular injury produced by alcohol results in a broad spectrum of clinical manifestations, ranging from relatively asymptomatic hepatomegaly to the development of massive steatonecrosis and fulminant hepatic failure.

TABLE 10–8. Signs of Alcoholic Hepatitis

| Sign | Frequency (%) |
| --- | --- |
| Hepatomegaly | 81–98 |
| Jaundice | 37–70 |
| Ascites | 32–76 |
| Fever | 28–65 |
| Malnutrition (wasting, weight loss) | 55 |
| Splenomegaly | 27–38 |
| Spider angioma | 22–65 |
| GI blood loss | 14–22 |
| Hepatic coma | 9–10 |
| Edema | 28–49 |
| Collateral venous pattern | 22 |

From Monroe PS, Baker AL: Alcoholic hepatitis. Postgrad Med 69:32, 1981.

2. Clinical assessment and risk
   a. Tables 10–8, 10–9, and 10–10 review the signs, symptoms, and laboratory findings of alcoholic hepatitis.
   b. Mikkelsen and co-workers have shown that the liver biopsy, laboratory data, and physical examination are significant as preoperative predictors of mortality.[7] In our experience, a thorough history, physical examination, and laboratory assessment are sufficient; liver

TABLE 10–9. Symptoms of Alcoholic Hepatitis

| Symptom | Frequency (%) |
| --- | --- |
| Anorexia | 77–100 |
| Weakness | 77–100 |
| Nausea and vomiting | 50–77 |
| Abdominal pain | 45–62 |
| Weight loss | 43–59 |
| Diarrhea | 12–27 |
| Jaundice | 8–13 |
| Hematemesis | 4 |

From Monroe PS, Baker AL: Alcoholic hepatitis. Postgrad Med 69:32, 1981.

**TABLE 10–10. Laboratory Findings in Alcoholic Hepatitis**

| Finding | Frequency (%) |
|---|---|
| SGOT | |
|   Normal | 9–15 |
|   Elevated | 89–91 |
|   Markedly elevated (> 300 IU/liter) | 5 |
| Elevated SGPT | 35–48 |
| Elevated bilirubin | 59–94 |
| Elevated alkaline phosphatase | 62–82 |
| Prolonged prothrombin time | 60 |
| Decreased albumin | 53–60 |
| Anemia | 43–70 |
| Leukocytosis | 35–60 |

From Monroe PS, Baker AL: Alcoholic hepatitis. Postgrad Med 69:32, 1981.

    biopsy is rarely indicated. Findings are shown in Tables 10–11 and 10–12.
- c. Cohen and Kaplan used the SGOT/SGPT ratio to diagnose patients with alcoholic hepatitis when the SGOT and SGPT were less than 300 units.[8] A ratio of greater than two was found in 70 per cent of patients with alcoholic hepatitis.
- d. Laboratory studies
  - (1) CBC with platelets
  - (2) Electrolytes, BUN, glucose
  - (3) Creatinine
  - (4) Prothrombin time and partial thromboplastin time
  - (5) SGOT, SGPT, alkaline phosphatase, bilirubin, albumin
  - (6) Amylase
  - (7) Urinalysis
  - (8) ECG
  - (9) Chest x-ray

## B. PERIOPERATIVE MANAGEMENT

1. Thiamine 100 mg PO once a day
2. Multivitamins T PO once a day
3. Improve nutritional status.
4. If prothrombin is abnormal, it must be corrected preoperatively (see section on cirrhosis).
5. If the patient is encephalopathic, this condition must be treated (see section on cirrhosis).

**TABLE 10–11. Signs and Laboratory Findings**

| Data | Deaths (12) | Survivors (11) |
|---|---|---|
| History | | |
|   Age, mean (range) | 51 (29–65) | 54 (37–75) |
|   Sex, male/female | 3/5 | 9/2 |
|   Race, Caucasian/Negro | 12/0 | 10/1 |
|   Alcoholism | 11 (1  ?) | 10 (1  ?) |
| Physical examination | | |
|   Encephalopathy | 10 | 2 |
|   Ascites | 12 | 2 |
|   Jaundice | 12 | 4 |
|   Fever over 100°F. | 10 | 6 |
|   Hepatomegaly | 11 | 10 |
|   Liver tenderness | 7 | 6 |
| Laboratory | | |
|   White blood cells in 1000's, mean (range) | 19.8 (10.7–36) | 9.0 (5.4–14.7) |
|   Bilirubin (mg %), mean (range) | 13.1 (1.4–36) | 2.5 (0.7–9.9) |
|   Albumin (gm %), mean (range) | 2.5 (1.2–3.5) | 3.4 (2.1–1.9) |
|   Prothrombin (%), mean (range) | 45 (13–82) | 74 (40–100) |
|   SGOT, mean (range) | 114 (57–220) | 106 (16–273) |
|   SGPT, mean (range) | 28 (19–36) | 29 (7–60) |
| Histologic evidence of cirrhosis | 12 | 7 |

From Harville DD, Summerskill WH: Surgery in acute hepatitis. JAMA *184*:4, 1963.

**TABLE 10–12. Liver Biopsy***

| Morphologic Appearance of Hyaline | Deaths (12) | Survivors (11) |
|---|---|---|
| Group I: Coarsely granular hyaline material without large discrete clumps | 0 | 2 |
| Group II: Irregular hyaline meshwork or masses | 1 | 3 |
| Group III: Rounded or discrete intracytoplasmic hyaline bodies (classic Mallory bodies) | 11 | 4 |

*Comparison of morphologic appearance of intracellular hyaline in survivors and those dying among twenty-three patients with acute hyaline necrosis who did not have a portacaval shunt

From Mikkelsen WP, Turrill FL, Kern WH: Acute hyaline necrosis of the liver. Am J Surg *116*:266, 1968.

## VII. DRUG-INDUCED HEPATITIS

### A. PREOPERATIVE EVALUATION

1. Background and purpose

    Hepatic injury may follow exposure to or ingestion, either parenteral or inhalation, of a number of agents. Some authors divide this on the basis of histopathology (see Table 10–13), but we find it easier to consider the mechanism (see Table 10–14). One type of mechanism, the direct toxic effect, occurs with predictable regularity in exposed individuals and is dose-dependent. Two classic examples of this are acetaminophen and carbon tetrachloride. The second type of drug effect is the idiosyncratic reaction, which usually occurs infrequently and is unpredictable. The response is not dose-dependent and may appear at any time during or shortly after exposure. Examples of this are halothane, chlorpromazine, and oral contraceptives.

    The consultant's assessment is aimed at identifying the drugs being taken and the degree of hepatic involvement.

2. Clinical assessment

    a. Harville and Summerskill[6] evaluated 16 patients with drug-induced hepatitis who underwent surgery, and found no serious complications or mortality. We recommend removal of the drug and serial evaluation of liver function tests.

    b. Laboratory studies

        (1) CBC with platelets
        (2) Electrolytes, BUN, and glucose
        (3) Creatinine
        (4) SGOT, SGPT, alkaline phosphatase, bilirubin, albumin
        (5) Prothrombin time and partial thromboplastin time
        (6) Urinalysis
        (7) Chest x-ray
        (8) ECG
        (9) Toxicology screen on specific drug level

### B. PERIOPERATIVE MANAGEMENT

1. The offending drug is identified and removed.
2. In acetaminophen-induced hepatitis, acetylcysteine given by mouth or by nasogastric tube is effective in detoxification if instituted within the first 10 to 12 hours after ingestion.[9, 10]

    a. 140 mg/kg/body weight loading dose
    b. 70 mg/kg/body weight q4h for three days

**TABLE 10–13. Histopathology of Drug-Induced Hepatitis**

| | Direct Toxic Effect | | Idiosyncratic | | | Other |
|---|---|---|---|---|---|---|
| Features | CARBON TETRA-CHLORIDE, E.G. | ACETAMINO-PHEN, E.G. | HALOTHANE, E.G. | ISONIAZID, E.G. | CHLOR-PROMAZINE E.G. | ORAL CONTRACEPTIVE AGENTS, E.G. |
| Predictable and dose-related toxicity | + | + | 0 | 0 | 0 | + |
| Latent period | Short | Short | Variable | Variable | Variable | Variable |
| Arthralgia, fever, rash, eosinophilia | 0 | 0 | + | 0 | + | 0 |
| Liver morphology | Necrosis, fatty infiltration | Centrilobular necrosis | Similar to viral hepatitis | Similar to viral hepatitis | Cholestasis *with* portal inflammation | Cholestasis *without* portal inflammation |

From Dienstag JL, Wands JR, Koff RS: Acute hepatitis, in Thorn GN et al (eds): Harrison's Principles of Internal Medicine, 9th ed. New York, McGraw-Hill, 1980, p 1467.

**TABLE 10–14. Toxic and Drug-Induced Hepatic Injury***

| Principal Morphologic Change | Class of Agent | Example |
|---|---|---|
| Cholestasis | Anabolic steroid | Methyl testosterone† |
| | Antithyroid | Methimazole |
| | Chemotherapeutic | Erythromycin estolate |
| | Oral contraceptive | Norethynodrel with mestranol |
| | Oral hypoglycemic | Chlorpropamide† |
| | Tranquilizer | Chlorpromazine† |
| Fatty liver | Chemotherapeutic | Tetracycline |
| Hepatitis | Anesthetic | Halothane‡ |
| | Anticonvulsant | Phenytoin |
| | Antihypertensive | α-Methyldopa† |
| | Chemotherapeutic | Isoniazid‡ |
| | Diuretic | Chlorothiazide |
| | Laxative | Oxyphenisatin‡ |
| Toxic (necrosis) | Hydrocarbon | Carbon tetrachloride |
| | Metal | Yellow phosphorus |
| | Mushroom | *Amanita phalloides* |
| | Analgesic | Acetaminophen |

*Principal alterations of hepatic morphology produced by some commonly used drugs and chemicals.

†Rarely associated with primary biliary cirrhosis.

‡Occasionally associated with chronic active hepatitis or submassive hepatic necrosis and cirrhosis.

# VIII. ISCHEMIC HEPATITIS

## A. PREOPERATIVE EVALUATION

1. Background and purpose

Another form of parenchymal liver cell injury results from impairment of normal cardiac function and can be classified as either congestive injury or ischemic hepatic injury. The significance is important, since the latter can mimic acute viral hepatitis with anorexia, malaise, jaundice, tender hepatomegaly, marked elevation in transaminase, and minimal elevation in alkaline phosphatase. Congestive injury rarely demonstrates these findings, and the transaminases are never greater than five times normal.[11] The factors that account for the differences in the two clinical pictures are that ischemic injury is predominantly a failure of liver perfusion (e.g., low cardiac output), whereas congestive injury is caused by venous congestion. In the preoperative assessment of such patients, the decreased blood flow secondary to anesthesia must be kept in mind, since liver injury could be exacerbated.

2. Clinical assessment
   a. Patients with hepatic congestion injury are at higher risk to progress to centrilobular necrosis if hypotension of hypoxemia should develop during surgery.
   b. Laboratory studies
      (1) CBC with platelets
      (2) Electrolytes, BUN, and glucose
      (3) SGOT, SGPT, alkaline phosphatase, bilirubin, albumin
      (4) Prothrombin time and thromboplastin time
      (5) ECG
      (6) Chest x-ray

## B. PERIOPERATIVE MANAGEMENT

1. In hepatic congestion, the goal is to return the patient to normal cardiac compensation. Caution should be taken to prevent too vigorous a diuresis, which could result in hypotension and ischemic injury.
2. Both ischemic and hepatic congestion will improve with observation and correction of the precipitating factors.
3. The prothrombin time should be corrected by the methods noted in the section on cirrhosis.
4. Drugs that undergo hepatic metabolism must be prescribed in such a way as to account for the degree of hepatic dysfunction.

## IX. CHOLESTATIC LIVER DISEASE

## A. PREOPERATIVE EVALUATION

1. Background and purpose
   This is a broad category of liver disease encompassing those entities that impair secretion of bile. Biochemically, this process is characterized by an increase in direct reacting bilirubin, alkaline phosphatase, gamma glutamyl transpeptidase, and serum bile acids. The thorough evaluation of etiology for cholestasis is critical preoperatively (see Table 10–15 to 10–17). The second important aspect is to manage the sequelae of hyperbilirubinemia pre- and postoperatively.

**TABLE 10–15. Causes of Extrahepatic Biliary Obstruction**

| | |
|---|---|
| Choledocholithiasis | 40% |
| Pancreatic cancer | 20% |
| Cholangiocarcinoma | 17% |
| Ampulla of Vater carcinoma, tumors of the porta hepatitis | 3% |
| Common duct obstruction other than stones (bile duct stricture, papillary stenosis, pancreatic pseudocysts, sclerosis, cholangitis) | 20% |

Adapted from Cello JP: Diagnostic approaches to jaundice. Hosp Pract, February 1982, p 49.

**TABLE 10–16. Causes of Intrahepatic Biliary Obstruction**

Focal abscess, carcinoma, cysts, parasites

Intrahepatic biliary atresia

Suppurative and nonsuppurative cholangitis
—bacterial
—immunologic (primary biliary cirrhosis, inflammatory bowel disease)

From Cello JP: Diagnostic approaches to jaundice. Hosp Pract, February 1982, p 49.

**TABLE 10–17. Causes of Intrahepatic Cholestasis Without Anatomic Biliary Obstruction**

Virus
Alcohol
Drugs
Sepsis
Cholestasis of infancy
Recurrent jaundice of pregnancy
Postoperative cholestasis

From Cello JP: Diagnostic approaches to jaundice. Hosp Pract, February 1982, p 49.

2. Clinical assessment
   a. Prolonged prothrombin time: This results from impaired bile salt excretion into the intestine, leading to poor fat absorption and steatorrhea. The steatorrhea causes decreased absorption of vitamin K. This condition can be treated with supplemental parenteral vitamin K.
   b. Renal failure in obstructive jaundice: The incidence of this process has been reported by Dawson and Bailey.[12, 13] Dawson found the incidence of renal failure to be 6 per cent, with direct correlation between preoperative bilirubin and creatinine clearance postoperatively. Bailey, on the other hand, confirmed the magnitude of postoperative renal failure in obstructive jaundice but could not document the linear effect of bilirubin and creatinine clearance.
   c. Laboratory studies
      (1) CBC with platelets
      (2) Electrolytes, BUN, glucose
      (3) Creatinine
      (4) Prothrombin time and partial thromboplastin time
      (5) SGOT, SGPT, alkaline phosphatase, bilirubin, albumin
      (6) Urinalysis
      (7) Chest x-ray
      (8) ECG

## B. Perioperative Management

1. An abnormal prothrombin time is corrected with vitamin K (see cirrhosis section).
2. Mannitol (10%) 500-ml infusion two hours before surgery and one bottle a day for two days. (Assessment of cardiac status before infusion is critical.)
3. See section on cholecystitis.

# X. CHRONIC ACTIVE HEPATITIS

## A. PREOPERATIVE EVALUATION

1. Background and purpose
   Chronic active hepatitic is a disorder characterized by continuing hepatic necrosis, active inflammation, and fibrosis leading to macronodular cirrhosis. Etiologies for the process are numerous (see Table 10–18). Probably the most common is infection with hepatitis B or non-A, non-B. The preoperative consultant must attempt to

**TABLE 10–18. Etiology of Chronic Active Hepatitis**

| Viral Hepatitis | Drug |
|---|---|
| Type B | Oxyphenisatin |
| Non-A, non-B | Methyldopa |
| Cytomegalovirus | Isoniazid |
| Rubella virus | Alcohol |
| Lupoid, or autoimmune, hepatitis | Aspirin, acetaminophen |

**Other**
Wilson's disease
Alpha$_1$-antitrypsin deficiency

Adapted from Sherlock S: Chronic hepatitis. Postgrad Med 65:81, 1979.

assess the etiology and correct the sequelae of the liver disease.

2. Clinical assessment and risk
   a. Chronic persistent hepatitis is a mild nonspecific hepatic inflammatory process that is self-limited and does not progress to cirrhosis. LaMont contends that, since this is a stable process, the anesthesia risk is low.[14]
   b. Two reports by Ward and associates and Boye and associates showed that surgery in chronic active hepatitis did not increase mortalilty and morbidity.[15, 16] The only report to the contrary was by Hargrove, who presented two patients with chronic active hepatitis and severe liver abnormalities who died postoperatively.[17] These reports are outlined in Table 10–19.
   c. The studies by Ward and associates and Boye and associates cited patients who had mildly elevated but stable liver function tests. Tests of Hargrove's two patients showed progressive liver failure at the time of surgery. We conclude from these reports that general anesthesia in the setting of progressive liver disease carries a higher risk than when liver function tests are stable.

**TABLE 10–19. Surgery in Chronic Active Hepatitis**

| Study | No. of Patients | Procedure | Mortality (%) |
|---|---|---|---|
| Ward et al. | 3 | Abdominal surgery | 0 |
| Boye et al. | 6 | Splenectomy | 0 |
| Hargrove | 2 | Laparotomy | 100 |

    d. Laboratory studies
       (1) CBC with platelets
       (2) Electrolytes, BUN, and glucose
       (3) Serum albumin
       (4) SGOT, SGPT, alkaline phosphatase, albumin
       (5) Bilirubin (total and direct)
       (6) ECG
       (7) Chest x-ray
       (8) Diagnostic evaluation of chronic active hepatitis should include $HB_sAg$, anti-$HB_c$, anti-$HB_s$, ceruloplasmin, antinuclear antibody, and liver biopsy (when indicated).

## B. PERIOPERATIVE MANAGEMENT

1. The following etiologies for chronic active hepatitis are listed with the recommended therapy.
    a. Drug-induced: discontinue agent
    b. Alcoholic disease: abstention
    c. Wilson's disease: penicillamine
    d. Alpha-$_1$-antitrypsin: no treatment
    e. Cytomegalovirus and rubella: no treatment
2. Lupoid, or autoimmune, hepatitis responds to steroids. Remission is induced in 80 per cent of patients on steroids within two to three years, although half of these will relapse after treatment is stopped, requiring retreatment.[18]
3. The efficacy of steroids in non-A, non-B chronic active hepatitis is not established. Most cases of chronic active hepatitis by hepatitis B do not respond to steroids.
4. If the patient is on steroid therapy, appropriate coverage for surgery is necessary (see Chapter 7 for details).
5. A prolonged prothrombin time is corrected with vitamin K and fresh frozen plasma (see cirrhosis section).

# XI. CIRRHOSIS

## A. PREOPERATIVE EVALUATION

1. Background and purpose
    Cirrhosis is a generic term that includes all forms of chronic diffuse liver disease. It is characterized by extensive loss of liver cells and by collapse and fibrosis of the supporting reticulin network, with distortion of the vascular bed and nodular regeneration of the remaining liver cell masses surrounded by fibrous tissue. The sine qua non of cirrhosis is extensive disorganization of the hepatic

**TABLE 10–20. Causes of Cirrhosis**

| |
|---|
| Alcohol |
| Primary biliary cirrhosis |
| Hemochromatosis |
| Sarcoidosis |
| Chlorpromazine |
| Chronic active hepatitis |
| • viral |
| • autoimmune |
| • drug-induced |
| • Wilson's disease |
| • alpha$_1$-antitrypsin deficiency |
| Postnecrotic |
| Cardiac |

lobular architecture. The various etiologies of cirrhosis are reviewed in Table 10–20. The approach of the preoperative consultant is to assess the sequelae of cirrhotic liver disease and estimate the degree of risk from these factors. Tables 10–21 to 10–23, compiled for alcoholic cirrhosis can be used for other etiologies as well.

2. Clinical assessment
   a. Deutsch showed that at least 85 per cent of patients with liver disease had at least one abnormal clotting test and only 15 per cent of patients had abnormal bleeding.[19]
   b. The coagulation abnormalities that accompany hepatocellar disease are as follows:
      (1) Decreased synthesis of clotting factors
      (2) Increased utilization of clotting factors
      (3) Production of abnormal clotting factors
      (4) Platelet abnormalities
   c. Laboratory studies
      (1) CBC with platelets
      (2) Electrolytes, BUN, glucose
      (3) Albumin, SGOT, SGPT, alkaline phosphatase, bilirubin (total and direct)
      (4) Prothrombin and partial thromboplastin time
      (5) Chest x-ray
      (6) ECG

**TABLE 10–21. Classification of Cirrhosis**

|  | Group A | Group B | Group C |
|---|---|---|---|
| Bilirubin (mg/100 ml) | < 2.0 | 2.0–3.0 | > 3.0 |
| Albumin (g/100 ml) | > 3.5 | 3.0–3.5 | < 3.0 |
| Ascites | None | Easily controlled | Poorly controlled |
| Encephalopathy | None | Mild | Advanced |
| Nutritional status | Excellent | Good | Poor |

From Child CG: The Liver and Portal Hypertension in Major Problems in Clinical Surgery. Philadelphia, WB Saunders, 1964.

## B. RISK ANALYSIS

1. Child[20] developed a classification of cirrhosis for prediction of mortality in patients undergoing portacaval shunts (Table 10–21). Stone[21] proposed that this classification could be used for any surgical procedure and listed the risks noted in Table 10–22.
2. A third classification, by Pugh and co-workers,[22] assigns points to various chemical and biochemical measurements, and risk for surgery is predicted from this grading (Table 10–23). Good risk is 5 to 6 points, moderate risk is 7 to 9 points, and poor risk is 10 to 15 points.

**TABLE 10–22. Basic Liver Functions and Operability**

| | |
|---|---|
| Class A | No limitations. |
| | Normal response to all operations. |
| | Normal ability of liver to regenerate. |
| Class B | Some limitation to liver function. |
| | Altered response to all operations but tolerated well if prepared preoperatively. |
| | Limited ability to regenerate new hepatic parenchyma so that all sizeable liver resections are contraindicated. |
| Class C | Severe limitations to liver function. |
| | Poor response to all operations regardless of preparatory efforts. |
| | Liver resection, no matter what the size, is contraindicated. |

From Stone HH: Preoperative and postoperative care. Surg Clin North Am 47:409, 1977.

**TABLE 10–23. Grading of Severity of Liver Disease**

| Clinical and Biochemical Measurements | Points Scored for Increasing Abnormality | | |
|---|---|---|---|
| | 1 | 2 | 3 |
| Encephalopathy (grade) | None | 1 and 2 | 3 and 4 |
| Ascites | Absent | Slight | Moderate |
| Bilirubin (mg per 100 ml) | 1–2 | 2–3 | > 3 |
| Albumin (g per 100 ml) | 3·5 | 2·8–3·5 | < 2·8 |
| Prothrombin time (sec. prolonged) for primary biliary cirrhosis:— | 1–4 | 4–6 | > 6 |
| Bilirubin (mg per 100 ml) | 1–4 | 4–10 | 10 |

From Pugh RNH, Murray-Lyen IM, Dawson JL, et al: Transection of the esophagus for bleeding esophageal varices. Br J Surg *60*:646, 1973.

3. A fourth classification by Wirthlin and associates[23] (Fig. 10–4) is directed to patients with cirrhosis and nonvariceal gastroduodenal bleeding. The predicted mortality is based on a five-point system shown in Figure 10–4.

## C. PERIOPERATIVE MANAGEMENT

1. Vitamin K preparations are reviewed in Table 10–24.[24–26]
2. Intravenous vitamin $K_1$ should be administered slowly, at a rate of approximately 10 mg per minute, well diluted in saline solution. There has been associated peripheral vascular collapse with intravenous use.
3. If rapid improvement in the coagulation status is necessary, fresh frozen plama is the preparation of choice. Table 10–25 lists parenteral blood products.[27] Spector and associates showed that the correction of a prolonged prothrombin time for emergency surgery or an invasive procedure requires volumes of fresh frozen plasma.[28] The results of this study show that the decay of factors II, VII, and IX is two to four hours; factor V is more variable. Repeated fresh frozen plasma transfusion is needed to maintain the improved prothrombin time.
4. Encephalopathy[29]
   a. Lactulose 30 ml PO until loose bowel movement, then q.i.d. or adjust to maintain bowel activity at three movements a day.
5. Goal of therapy: Loss of not more than 1 kg/day if both ascites and edema are present, or no more than 0.5 kg/day in patients with ascites only.

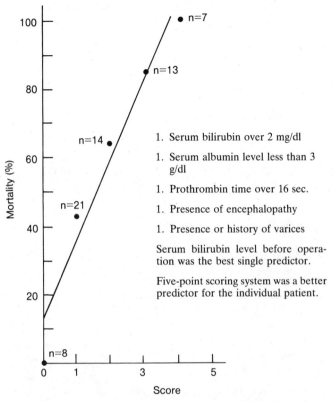

1. Serum bilirubin over 2 mg/dl

1. Serum albumin level less than 3 g/dl

1. Prothrombin time over 16 sec.

1. Presence of encephalopathy

1. Presence or history of varices

Serum bilirubin level before operation was the best single predictor.

Five-point scoring system was a better predictor for the individual patient.

**Figure 10–4.** Predicted mortality in cirrhosis of the liver and nonvariceal gastroduodenal bleeding, based on a five-point system.

**TABLE 10–24. Vitamin K Therapy in Cirrhosis**

| Type | Route | Dose | Action | Prothrombin Lab Eval. |
|------|-------|------|--------|------------------------|
| Fat-soluble AquaMephyton ($K_1$) | SC, IM, IV | 5–10 mg | 6–12 h | Check 12 h |
| Mephyton ($K_1$) | PO | 5–10 mg | 12–24 h | Check 24 h |
| Water-soluble Synkamin ($K_5$) | PO, SC, IM, IV | 1–5 mg | 12–24 h | Check 12 h |

**TABLE 10–25. Therapeutic Regimen to Improve Coagulation Status**

| Preparation | Factors | Volume | Dose | Risk |
|---|---|---|---|---|
| Fresh frozen plasma | All factors | 200–300 ml | 15–20 ml/kg, then one third the dose q6–8 h | Low risk |
| Konyne | II, VII, IX, X | 20–30 ml | | Hepatitis |
| Proplex | II, VII, IX, X | 20–30 ml | | Hepatitis |

    a. Bed rest and strict fluid and sodium restrictions
    b. Spironolactone 25 mg PO q.i.d. (increase in increment, every four days to a maximum of 100 mg q.i.d)
    c. Furosemide 40 to 80 mg PO once a day

# REFERENCES

*Liver Disease*

1. Cooperman LH, Wollman H, Marsh ML: Anesthesia on the liver. Surg Clin North Am 57:421, 1977.
2. Batchelder BM, Cooperman LH: Effects of anesthesia on splanchnic circulation and metabolism. Surg Clin North Am 55:787, 1975.

*Viral Hepatitis*

3. Medical Knowledge Self-Assessment Program VI, Section Gastroenterology, American College of Physicians, Part I, 1982, p 43.
4. Dienstag JL, Wands JR, Koff RS: Acute hepatitis, in Thorn GW, et al (eds): Harrison's Principles of Internal Medicine, 9th ed. New York, McGraw-Hill, 1980, p 1459.
5. Bundell CR, Earnest DL: Medical evaluation of the patient with liver disease prior to surgery, in Brown BR (ed): Anesthesia and the Patient with Liver Disease. Philadelphia, FA Davis, 1981, p 123.
6. Harville DD, Summerskill WH: Surgery in acute hepatitis. JAMA 184:4, 1963.

*Alcoholic Liver Disease*

7. Mikkelsen WP, Turrill FL, Kern WH: Acute hyaline necrosis of the liver. Am J Surg 116:266, 1968.
8. Cohen JA, Kaplan MM: The SGOT/SGPT ratio—An indicator of alcoholic liver disease. Dig Dis Sci 24:835, 1979.

*Drug-induced Hepatitis*

9. Medical Knowledge Self-Assessment Program VI, Section Gastroenterology, American College of Physicians, Part I, 1983, p 7.
10. Peterson RG, Rumack BH: Treating acute acetaminophen poisoning with acetylcysteine. JAMA 237:2406, 1977.

*Ischemic Hepatitis*

11. Bynum TE, Boitnatt JK, Maddrey WC: Ischemic hepatitis. Dig Dis Sci *24*:129, 1979.

*Cholestatic Liver Disease*

12. Dawson JL: The incidence of postoperative renal failure in obstructive jaundice. Br J Surg *52*:663, 1965.
13. Bailey ME: Endotoxin, bile salts, and renal function in obstructive jaundice. Br J Surg *63*:774, 1976.

*Chronic Active Hepatitis*

14. LaMont JT: The liver. *In* Vandam LE (ed.): Making the Patient Ready for Surgery. Menlo Park, CA, Addison-Wesley Publishing Co., 1984, p. 47.
15. Ward ME, Adu-Gyame Y, Strunin L: Althesin and pancuranium in chronic liver disease. Anaesthesia *47*:1199, 1975.
16. Boye NP, Norday A, Gjone E: Splenectomy in chronic active hepatitis. Scand J Gastroenterol *7*:747, 1972.
17. Hargrove MD: Chronic active hepatitis: Possible adverse effects of exploratory laparotomy. Surgery *68*:771, 1970.
18. Wright EC, Seeff LB, Berk PD, Jones A, Plotz PH: Treatment of chronic active hepatitis: An analysis of three controlled trials. Gastroenterology *73*:1422, 1979.

*Cirrhosis*

19. Deutsch E: Blood coagulation changes in liver disease, in Popper H, Schaffner F (eds): Progress in Liver Diseases, vol. 2. New York, Grune & Stratton, 1965, pp 69–83.
20. Child CG: The Liver and Portal Hypertension in Major Problems in Clinical Surgery. Philadelphia, WB Saunders, 1964, p. 50.
21. Stone HH: Preoperative and postoperative care. Surg Clin North Am *47*:409, 1977.
22. Pugh RNH, Murray-Lyen IM, Dawson JL, et al: Transection of the esophagus for bleeding esophageal varices. Br J Surg *60*:646, 1973.
23. Wirthlin LS, Urk HV, Malt RB, et al: Predictors of surgical mortality in patients with cirrhosis and non-variceal gastroduodenal bleeding. Surg Gynecol Obstet *139*:65, 1974.
24. Frick PG, Riedler G, Brogli H: Dose response and minimal daily requirement of vitamin K in month. J Appl Physiol *23*:387, 1967.
25. Deykin D: Warfare therapy (Part II). N Engl J Med *23*:801, 1970.
26. Shoskes M, Rothfield EL, Jacobs M: Colloidally suspended phytonadione in bishydroxycoumarin-induced hypoprothrombinemia. Am J Cardiol *8*:72, 1961.
27. Buchanan GR: Hemophilia. Pediatr Clin North Am *27*:309, 1980.
28. Spector I, Corn M, Tickten HE: Effect of plasma transfusion on the prothrombin time and clotting factors in liver disease. N Engl J Med *275*:1032, 1966.
29. Perrillo RP: Liver disease. *In* Freitag JJ, Miller LW (eds.): Manual of Medical Therapeutics, 23rd ed. Boston, Little, Brown and Co., 1980, Chap. 12, p. 248.

# THE RENAL SYSTEM: FLUID AND ELECTROLYTE DISORDERS; KIDNEY DISEASE

## I. FLUID BALANCE

### A. PREOPERATIVE EVALUATION

1. Purpose

   Any abnormality of fluid balance will increase the operative risk and should be corrected whenever possible. The amount of time available and therefore the amount of correction that can be done depends on the emergency of the surgery. Sometimes delaying surgery will exacerbate the problems, and incomplete correction must be accepted.

2. Clinical assessment

   a. Basics of water balance

   (1) Body water and compartments: Sixty per cent of an adult's body weight is water. Of this, two thirds is in the intracellular space and one third is in the extracellular space. Of the extracellular water, three fourths is interstitial fluid and one fourth is intravascular fluid. Another way to look at this is that intracellular fluid is 8/12, interstitial is 3/12, and intravascular is 1/12 of total body water. This is summarized in Figure 11–1.

   (2) Volume distribution; osmotic and hydrostatic forces: Distribution of water between body compartments depends on balance of the hydrostatic versus the osmotic forces.

   (3) Intracellular space: Osmotic forces of the intracellular space are determined by intracellular protein, potassium, and chloride.

   (4) Extracellular space: The osmotic forces of the

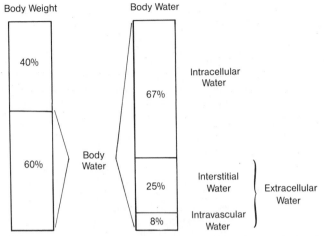

**Figure 11–1.** Distribution of body water in relation to total body weight.

extracellular fluid are principally the concentration of sodium, chloride, and bicarbonate. There is a free exchange of sodium chloride and bicarbonate ions and water between the interstitial and intravascular space. Serum proteins in the intravascular space provide an inward osmotic force counterbalancing the outward hydrostatic forces.

Any disruption of these forces by a reduction in serum proteins, elevation in capillary pressure, or disruption in capillary wall function will cause fluid shifts between the compartments.

(5) Intravascular space: Low intravascular volume (dehydration) decreases tissue perfusion and may result in organ injury. Even minor dehydration can decrease renal blood flow during surgery, resulting in acute necrosis, although the blood pressure remains selectively normal. Signs of dehydration are poor tissue turgor, dry mucous membranes, and reduced sweating.

An expanded intravascular volume may result from cardiac, renal, or hepatic failure. Inadequate organ perfusion may be present in some edematous disorders, such as congestive heart failure, even though the intravascular volume is increased or normal.

(6) Distribution of intravenous fluids and electrolytes

    (a) Water: Because of its rapid exchange with other compartments, water by itself is ineffective in expanding the intravascular volume.

    (b) Saline: saline solution rapidly expands the intravascular space, but three fourths of the administered solution quickly redistributes to the interstitium.

    (c) Albumin: Albumin in solutions is valuable in expanding the intravascular volume. However, in most hypoalbuminemic states the rapid catabolism of the albumin and the poor reduction owing to underlying disease allows the administered albumin to be only transiently helpful.

    (d) Blood: Whole blood rapidly expands the intravascular volume but is indicated only in acute or chronic blood loss with absolute deficiency of red blood cells.

b. Evaluating the state of hydration

(1) History: Dehydration frequently results from nausea or vomiting, prolonged fasting—perhaps in preparation for surgery—fever, diarrhea, or inability to drink. Overhydration is frequently seen with chronic liver failure, congestive heart failure, nephrotic syndrome, and iatrogenic fluid overload. Acute renal failure causes fluid overload because of sudden drop of output.

Table 11–1 summarizes clinical and laboratory clues to abnormal hydration.

A review of the patient's charts may reveal evidence of abnormal hydration. The review should include the anesthesia record, which shows blood loss as well as intraoperative fluid replacement in a patient who has had previous surgery.

A careful record of the patient's weight is invaluable. Other clues include a change in blood pressure and unbalanced intake/output.

(2) Physical examination: Physical evidence of dehydration includes thirst, weakness, apathy, absence of groin and axillary sweat, poor tissue turgor, and dry mucous membranes. Pronounced intravascular volume reduction causes orthostatic hypotension, a resting tachycardia, cool extremities,

**TABLE 11–1. Clues to Dehydration**

| | History | Chart Data | Lab Data | Physical Signs |
|---|---|---|---|---|
| Total body and vascular depletion | Nasogastric suction<br>Nausea or vomiting<br>NPO for surgery<br>Fever<br>Diarrhea<br>Unable to drink<br>Bleeding | Intake/output (including meals)<br>↓ BP ↑ Pulse<br>Weight loss | Serum sodium ↑ or ↓<br>Hemoglobin ↑<br>BUN/creatinine > 20<br>Urine sodium < 10 mEq/L<br>Urine specific gravity > 1.015 | Orthostatic hypotension<br>Low blood pressure<br>Weak pulse<br>Neck veins flat<br>Poor skin turgor<br>Dry mucous membranes<br>Thirst, weakness<br>Apathy, syncope, coma |
| Total body normal or excess fluid with vascular depletion | Tissue trauma<br>Burn<br>Liver disease<br>Nephrosis<br>Heart failure | Weight gain | Not helpful | Edema<br>Distended neck veins and rales in heart failure |

weak pulse, and reduced urine volume. The percentage of dehydration may be estimated roughly as follows: 2%, thirst; 5%, loss of axillary sweat; 10%, postural hypotension in absence of other causes.

Evidence of overhydration includes edema, ascites, physical signs of heart failure, such as an $S_3$ gallop, pulmonary rales, and an elevated jugular venous pressure.

(3) Laboratory data: Laboratory data are an adjunct to the clinical evaluation of the patient. They must be interpreted in light of the patient's history and physical examination.

Except in unusual circumstances of excessive salt administration, hypernatremia indicates dehydration. An increased or rising hemoglobin suggests dehydration. A change in the BUN to serum creatinine ratio from a normal of 10 to 1 to a higher level also suggests dehydration, as does an increased urine specific gravity.

*Caution:* False elevations of the urine specific gravity are seen when other osmotic particles, such as glucose or radiocontrast dyes, are present in the urine. Urine sodium excretion will be low in a dehydrated patient with good intrinsic renal function unless the patient is taking diuretics.

## B. RISK ESTIMATION

It is difficult to develop a numerical risk estimation based on fluid or electrolyte abnormalities alone, as these are often related to underlying disease.

## C. ETIOLOGIES OF FLUID IMBALANCE

1. Dehydration
   a. Fever
   b. Inadequate intake
   c. Sweating
   d. Diuretic therapy
   e. Vomiting and diarrhea
2. Overhydration
   a. Acute renal failure
   b. Congestive heart failure
   c. Overuse of IV fluids
   d. Liver failure
   e. Aortic aneurysm

## II. ELECTROLYTE DISORDERS

### A. PREOPERATIVE EVALUATION

1. Purpose: To review electrolytes with respect to etiology and management of the hypo and hyper states. The consultant must assess these abnormalities and attempt to correct the process before surgery.
2. Clinical assessment
   a. Sodium
      (1) Hypernatremia
         (a) The causes of hypernatremia are related to the status of the extracellular fluid volume. This is reviewed in Figure 11–2.
         (b) Confusion, somnolence, and coma are associated with hypernatremia. The severity of symptoms depend on the rate of change and absolute level of plasma sodium.
      (2) Hyponatremia
         (a) As with hypernatremia, the causes of hyponatremia are related to the extracellular fluid volume. Figure 11–3 reviews the etiologies.
         (b) Confusion, somnolence, seizures, and coma are symptoms of hyponatremia. The severity of these symptoms depends on the rate of change of plasma sodium; they rarely occur above a serum sodium of 115 mEq/L.
   b. Potassium
      (1) Hyperkalemia
         (a) Elevation in serum potassium results from four mechanisms, as shown in Figure 11–4:
         (b) Weakness, fatigue, confusion, numbness, and tingling are common symptoms of hyperkalemia.
         (c) Cardiac dysfunction is the most life-threatening aspect of elevated serum potassium. Table 11–2 is a correlation of serum potassium and ECG changes.
      (2) Hypokalemia
         (a) A reduction in the serum potassium is secondary to three possible sources (Fig. 11–5):
         (b) Symptoms are due to impaired neuromuscular transmission with weakness, paralysis, and intestinal dilatation.
         (c) The most significant concern is the cardiac dysrhythmias and conduction defects associated with hypokalemia (Table 11–3).

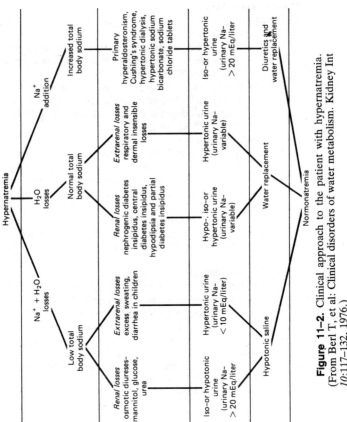

**Figure 11-2.** Clinical approach to the patient with hypernatremia. (From Berl T, et al: Clinical disorders of water metabolism. Kidney Int *10*:117–132, 1976.)

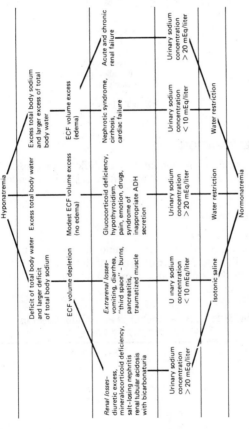

**Figure 11–3.** Causes of hyponatremia. (From Berl T, et al: Clinical disorders of water metabolism. Kidney Int *10*:117–132, 1976.)

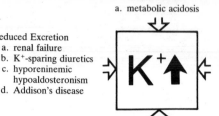

Redistribution
a. metabolic acidosis

Reduced Excretion
a. renal failure
b. $K^+$-sparing diuretics
c. hyporeninemic
   hypoaldosteronism
d. Addison's disease

Excess Input
a. potassium
   supplements
b. salt substitutes
c. rhabdomyolysis

Pseudohyperkalemia
a. leukocytosis
b. thrombocytosis
c. hemolysis

**Figure 11–4.**

## B. RISK ESTIMATION

Numerical estimation of risk is difficult to assess, since electrolyte abnormalities are often related to underlying disease.

## C. MANAGEMENT

1. Hypernatremia
   a. Calculate the water volume to correct the serum sodium to 150 mEq/L over 48 hours. Give only one half this amount in the first 24 hours.

**TABLE 11–2. Relationship of Potassium Level to Electrocardiographic Changes**

| Potassium mEq/L | ECG Change* |
|---|---|
| 5.5–7.5 | Peaked T waves |
| 7.5–9 | Flattening and widening of P wave, prolonged PR interval, reduced R wave, some widening of QRS |
| 9–10 | P wave disappears, widened QRS, decreased amplitude of T waves, verticular tachycardia, atrial fibrillation |
| 10 and above | Wide QRS, sine wave, ventricular standstill |

*Effect depends on serum concentration and rapidity of development.
Adapted from Feldman MS, Helfant RH: Disturbances of electrolyte balance, in Helfant RH (ed): Bellet's Essentials of Cardiac Arrhythmias. Philadelphia, WB Saunders, 1980.

**TABLE 11–3. Literature on Dysrhythmias and Conduct Defects Associated with Hypokalemia**

| Type | Reference |
|------|-----------|
| U wave | Feldman & Helfant[1] |
| Sinus bradycardia | Chung[2] |
| Junctional and atrial tachycardia with block | Davidson & Surawicz[3] |
| Ventricular fibrillation | Kunin, Surawicz, & Simr[4] |
| Potentiation of the arrhythmic effects of digitalis | Surawicz & Gettes[5] |

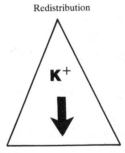

Redistribution

Reduced Intake                     Losses

Redistribution                     Reduced Intake

  a. alkalosis                    a. alcoholism
  b. insulin infusion            b. anorexia nervosa
                                   c. starvation

Losses

a. Urinary
  1. mineralocorticoid
    a. aldosteronism
    b. Cushing's syn-
      drome
    c. Bartter's syn-
      drome
  2. renal wasting
    a. RTA
    b. diuretics
  3. antibiotics
    a. amphotericin B
    b. carbenicillin

b. G.I.
  1. stomach
    a. nasogastric suc-
      tioning
    b. vomiting
  2. fistula
  3. biliary drainage
  4. diarrhea
  5. ureterosigmoidos-
    tomy

c. Skin
  1. sweating

**Figure 11–5.**

### TABLE 11–4. Replacement Therapy for Hypernatremia

| Etiology | Replacement | |
|---|---|---|
| $Na^+ + H_2O$ losses | 0.45% | NaCl |
| | 0.5% | NaCl |
| | 0.9% | NaCl |
| $H_2O$ losses | 5% | D/W |
| $Na^+$ addition | 5% | D/W + diuretics |

Body water deficit = normal total body water − current total body water

$$BWD = NTBW - CTBW$$

$$= NTBW - \frac{\text{normal } Na^+ \times NTBW}{\text{measured } Na^+}$$

$$= NTBW \left( 1 - \frac{\text{normal } Na^+}{\text{measured } Na^+} \right)$$

$$= NTBW \left( \frac{\text{measured } Na^+ - \text{normal } Na^+}{\text{measured } Na^+} \right)$$

$$= 0.6 \times \frac{\text{normal body}}{\text{weight (kg)}} \left( \frac{\text{measured } Na^+ - \text{normal } Na^+}{\text{measured } Na^+} \right)$$

    b. Fluid therapy (see Table 11–4):
    c. Check serum $Na^+$ every six hours.
  2. Hyponatremia
    a. The amount of sodium required to raise the sodium to a desired level can be calculated from the following formula:

mEq Na required = body weight (kg) × 0.6 (L/kg) × (desired $Na^+$ − observed $Na^+$)

    b. Fluid therapy (see Table 11–5):

### TABLE 11–5. Replacement Therapy for Hyponatremia

| Etiology | Replacement |
|---|---|
| Deficit of total body water and larger deficit of total body sodium | 0.9% NaCl = 154 mEq/L<br>3% NaCl = 513 mEq/L |
| Excess total body water | Water restriction |
| Excess total body sodium and larger excess of total body water | Water restriction |

    c. Replace the $Na^+$ gradually, checking the serum $Na^+$ every six hours.

    d. If symptoms are severe, use the 3% NaCl solution slowly and cautiously. Follow the cardiac status in the elderly population very closely. Watch $K^+$ carefully; large $Na^+$ load presented to distal tubules can result in rapid $K^+$ loss.

3. Hyperkalemia
    a. The approach to management is directed at three aspects, depending on the degree of hyperkalemia, the ECG findings, and the clinical status of the patient. The three approaches are as follows:
      (1) Antagonize the effects of $K^+$
      (2) Force $K^+$ into the cells
      (3) Remove $K^+$ from the body
    b. Antagonize the effects of $K^+$
      (1) When the serum $K^+$ is above 8 mEq/L, or ECG changes are present (see Table 11–2), we initiate therapy as follows:
        (a) Cardiac monitor
        (b) Calcium gluconate 10 ml of 10% solution IV over two minutes. This may be repeated in five minutes.
        (c) The duration of action of calcium gluconate is approximately 1 hour.
        (d) Following calcium gluconate use therapies c and d.
    c. Force $K^+$ into the cells.
      (1) When the serum $K^+$ is greater than 8 mEq/L and therapy has been initiated as above, we begin the following regimen:
        (a) Sodium bicarbonate ($NaHCO_3$) one ampul IV over five minutes. This may be repeated in 10 to 15 minutes. Duration of action is one to two hours. (Don't mix $HCO_3$ and $Ca^{++}$.)
        (b) Dextrose (D50) one ampul IV over five minutes plus 5 to 10 units of regular insulin IV. Duration of action is several hours.
        (c) Dextrose (D10) + sodium bicarbonate + regular insulin. A solution of 1000 ml D10 and water with two ampuls of sodium bicarbonate is infused at 300 ml/hour over the first 30 minutes and the remainder over three hours. Twenty-five units of regular insulin is given subcutaneously. Duration of action is several

hours. This method should be used with caution in patients with limited cardiac reserve.

d. Remove $K^+$ from the body.
   (1) When the serum $K^+$ is greater than 6 mEq/L, we initiate therapy as follows:
      (a) Kayexalate
         *(1)* Oral administration: 50 gm in 200 ml of 20% sorbitol. This is given every six hours until the $K^+$ is normal.
         *(2)* Rectal administration: 50 gm plus 50 gm sorbitol in 200 ml water as a retention enema (30 to 60 minutes). This is repeated every hour until the $K^+$ is normal.
      (b) Renal dialysis
      (c) Fludrocortisone acetate (Florinef) 0.1 mg/day in patients with hyporeninemic hypoaldosteronism (type IV renal tubular acidosis).

4. Hypokalemia
   a. Elective or emergency surgery ($K^+$ 2.8–3.5 mEq/L)

   *Intravenous* (level between 2.8–3 mEq/L)
   30 mEq in a saline solution at 10 mEq/h. Check $K^+$ in 12 h (using IVAC).
   *Oral* (level between 3–3.5 mEq/L)
   10% KCl (20 mEq $K^+$) PO q8h or q12h. Check $K^+$ in 24 h.

   b. Elective surgery ($K^+$ 2.8 mEq/L)

   Postpone surgery and replace $K^+$ orally.

   c. Emergency surgery ($K^+$ 2.8 mEq/L)

   . *Intravenous* (central line, IVAC)
   Moderate (level between 2.8–2 mEq/L)
   40 mEq/L in a saline solution at 20 mEq/h. Check $K^+$ q6h until corrected.
   Severe (level <2 mEq/L)
   60 mEq in a saline solution at 40 mEq/h. Check $K^+$ after 120 mEq have been infused and q6h thereafter until the $K^+$ is corrected.

## REFERENCES

### *Electrolyte Disorders*

1. Feldman MS, Helfant RH: Disturbances of electrolyte balance, in Helfant RH: Bellet's Essentials of Cardiac Arrhythmias, 2nd ed. Philadelphia, WB Saunders, 1980, p 276.
2. Chung EK: Electrocardiographic findings in hypokalemia. Postgrad Med *51*:285, 1978.
3. Davidson S, Surawicz B: Ectopic beats and atrioventricular conduction disturbances in patients with hypopotassemia. Arch Intern Med *120*:280, 1976.
4. Kunin AS, Surawicz B, Simr EAH: Decrease in serum potassium concentrations and appearance of cardiac arrhythmias during infusion of potassium with glucose in potassium depleted patients. N Engl J Med *266*:228, 1962.
5. Surawicz B, Gettes LS: Effects of electrolyte abnormalities on the heart and circulation, in Conn HZ, Horowitz D (eds): Cardiac and Vascular Disease. Philadelphia, Lea & Febiger, 1971, Ch 21, p 539.

## III. RENAL DISEASE

## A. PREOPERATIVE EVALUATION

1. Purpose
   a. To determine level of renal function and etiology of disease
   b. To correct any reversible contributers to renal impairment and restore metabolic balance
   c. To prevent deterioration of renal function during surgery by strict monitoring of patient's status during the perioperative period
   d. To identify drugs given perioperatively that require modified dosage schedules owing to renal impairment
2. Clinical assessment
   a. History and physical examination
      (1) Determine whether there is a known history of renal disease.
      (2) Question patient concerning symptoms of urinary tract dysfunction, for example, dysuria, hematuria, infections, hesitancy, frequent or very infrequent urination.
      (3) Other clinical manifestations of renal disease are protean and may affect all organ systems. However, they are, for the most part, nonspecific and may be due to other problems. Common findings include:

- (a) Cardiovascular: Hypertension, congestive heart failure, pericarditis
- (b) Gastrointestinal: Nausea, vomiting, anorexia, constipation
- (c) Hematologic: Anemia, bleeding, infections
- (d) Endocrine: Hyperlipidemia, glucose intolerance, euthyroid "sick" syndrome

b. Laboratory assessment
  - (1) Renal function is evaluated in terms of glomerular and tubular components.
    - (a) Glomerular function
      - *(1)* Determined by analysis of creatinine clearance where

glomerular filtration rate (GFR) =

creatinine clearance (Ccr) = $\dfrac{UcrV}{Pcr}$

Where Ucr = urine creatinine concentration

V = urine flow rate

Pcr = plasma creatine concentration

Normal for males is in the range of 120 ml/minute, or 180 L/day, and about 85 per cent of this for women.

  - *(2)* Creatinine alone can also be used as a rough estimate of GFR, with 1 mg/dl reflecting a normal average GFR. Because a doubling of creatinine (to 2 mg/dl) indicates a 50 per cent decrease in GFR, it can be seen that small increases in creatinine in the lower range may reflect a large decrease in GFR.
  - *(3)* BUN also reflects glomerular filtration but may be elevated out of proportion to serum creatinine because it is altered by many factors other than the GFR. A high BUN/creatinine ratio (greater than 20 to 1) may be due to:
    - *a)* Increased tubular reabsorption of urea due to:

      Prerenal azotemia: decreased urine flow rate secondary to decreased renal perfusion

      Postrenal azotemia: decreased urine flow rate secondary to obstructed urine flow

      *b)* Increased urea production
         Increased protein catabolism—internal
           bleeding, trauma, shock, steroids
         Increased protein intake

  (b) Tubular function
     *(1)* Determination of tubular function gener-
        ally follows glomerular function.
     *(2)* Urine concentrating ability as measured
        by specific gravity is the most sensitive
        test, but specific testing of tubular func-
        tion is rarely required preoperatively.

(2) Urinalysis
  (a) Urine sediment: Urine sediment is of great
     importance in detecting and diagnosing renal
     disease. Although complete differential diag-
     nosis is beyond the scope of this discussion,
     greater than 0 to 4 RBCs, 0 to 4 WBCs, or 0
     to 1 renal tubular cells per high power field is
     abnormal and requires preoperative evalua-
     tion. Red blood cell casts indicate glomerular
     disease; white blood cell casts, pyelonephritis
     and interstitial disease; WBC and RBC casts
     may be seen in active glomerulonephritis.
     Findings in acute tubular necrosis include
     WBC and RBC casts, as well as coarse gran-
     ular casts.
  (b) Protein
     *(1)* Normally, less than 50 mg of protein is
        excreted in the urine per 24 hours.
     *(2)* Although "dipstick" screening of urine
        protein depends on urine concentration,
        greater than 1+ should be evaluated by
        a 24-hour collection for protein.
     *(3)* Mild elevation above 50 mg may be seen
        in the febrile patient. However, greater
        than 500 mg/24 hours nearly always is an
        indicator of intrinsic renal disease, and
        greater than 2 gm/24 hours signifies glo-
        merular disease.

(3) Blood chemistry and metabolic abnormalities:
  Multiple metabolic abnormalities result from renal
  impairment. Such abnormalities, which include
  the following, must be evaluated and stabilized
  preoperatively:
  (a) $Na^+$: Hyponatremia (decreased urine diluting
     capacity)

(b) $K^+$: Hyperkalemia (decreased $K^+$ excretion)
(c) $H^+/HCO_3^-$: Metabolic acidosis (renal $HCO_3^-$ wasting and decreased ammonia production)
(d) $Ca^{++}$, P: Hypocalcemia/hyperphosphatemia (phosphorus retention, decreased effective vitamin D)
(e) BUN: Azotemia (reduced nitrogen excretion, increased catabolism)

## B. RISK ESTIMATION

1. Many of the factors noted above increase the risk of surgery aside from renal insufficiency per se.
2. With strict attention to the patient's perioperative status, chronic renal failure patients who are carefully managed can tolerate surgery with reasonable mortality. Representative statistics from several series are as follows:
   a. No perioperative deaths among 17 dialysis patients undergoing 26 procedures reported by Hata and co-workers.[1]
   b. Two deaths among 31 hemodialysis patients undergoing 40 elective and 9 emergency procedures reported by Brenowitz and associates.[2]
      A general idea of risk can be assessed from these and other studies, although no specific factors have been defined.
3. Risk for surgery is not likely to be increased if creatinine clearance is greater than 50 per cent normal (creatinine less than 2 per cent). However, actual level of function at which risk increases significantly has not been determined.

## C. PERIOPERATIVE MANAGEMENT

1. Renal insufficiency
   a. Preservation of remaining renal function is of paramount importance, and parameters of renal function must be monitored closely.
   b. Regulation of volume status is critical.
      (1) Mild to moderate renal impairment: These patients are most at risk for volume depletion because of impaired renal concentrating ability early in the course of renal insufficiency. Observe carefully and replace fluids as needed.
      (2) Severe renal insufficiency: These patients are at risk for volume overload and hyperkalemia. Monitor fluid balance carefully and dialyze if necessary. Consider Swan-Ganz monitoring.

    (3) Treat anemia, particularly in the elderly or in patients with vascular disease.
  c. Maintain nutrition.
  d. Adjust drug dosages as noted below, being particularly careful with sedatives.

2. Dialysis patients
  a. Several physiologic alterations that may cause surgical complications need to be considered in the dialysis patient. These include:
    (1) Uremic bleeding owing to platelet dysfunction
    (2) Hyperkalemia: $K^+$ >5.5 mEq/L may be considered a contraindication to general anesthesia.
    (3) Fluid overload with congestive heart failure and hypertension
    (4) Acid–base imbalance
    (5) Increased infection rate
    (6) Impaired wound healing owing to poor nutritional status and anemia
  b. Dialysis performed within 24 hours before surgery is the key to successful management and minimization of risks. Dialysis should be completed at least six hours before surgery to minimize any bleeding tendency as a result of heparin used during dialysis.[3] Benefits of preoperative dialysis include reduction of uremic bleeding tendency, control of hyperkalemia, reduction of fluid overload, and correction of acid–base imbalance.
  c. Additional maneuvers to reduce surgical risk in the dialysis patient include:
    (1) Restriction of protein and potassium in the diet for several days before surgery, as nitrogen and potassium loads will be increased postoperatively owing to catabolism.
    (2) Although chronic anemia is generally well tolerated, hematocrits should be raised to the 30% range for patients with cardiovascular disease and for the elderly.
    (3) Careful use of sedatives and neuromuscular blocking agents and modification of drug doses as noted below.
    (4) Careful observation for early symptoms of infection, such as hypotention, tachycardia, lethargy and confusion, worsening of parameters of uremia. Treatment should be instituted early with broad-spectrum antibiotics pending cultures. Despite optimal preparation for surgery, there is an increased incidence of postoperative infections in

dialysis patients, particularly wound infections and
pneumonia.[4]

3. Renal transplant patients

a. Potential problems in the transplant patient are related
to immunosuppression and steroid therapy.

b. No increased incidence of postoperative wound infection was found by Stuart and associates, however.[5]
Antibiotics are recommended only for potentially con-
taminated surgical fields (e.g., urologic manipulation)
and oral surgery. Otherwise, prophylactic antibiotics
are not recommended.

4. Modification of drug dosages: Many drugs given to the
patient with renal impairment must be modified in dosage
because of altered metabolism or excretion. Every routine
drug, as well as those instituted in the perioperative
period, must be checked for appropriate alteration in
dosing.[6]

## D. ACUTE RENAL FAILURE

Acute renal failure is defined as an abrupt onset of rising
serum creatinine associated with inability of the body to
excrete nitrogenous wastes.

A patient with a urine output level of less than 500 ml/24
hours is oliguric. A patient with anuria (less than 50 ml/24
hours) should be evaluated for postrenal obstruction, such
as blocked catheter or prostatic obstruction. Rapid, efficient
evaluation is imperative to prevent acute tubular necrosis
and resulting complications. Classic acute tubular necrosis
occurs when the 24-hour urine volume is less than 400 ml.

1. Acute renal failure may be divided into prerenal, postrenal, and intrinsic renal causes (see Table 11–6).

a. Prerenal acute renal failure: Acute renal failure is said
to be prerenal if the kidney is inadequately perfused.
Dehydration caused by vomiting, diarrhea, and diuretics is the major cause.

b. Acute intrinsic renal failure: Acute intrinsic renal
failure is the result of renal injury. Although the
causes of acute intrinsic renal failure are varied, in the
surgical setting, a large percentage of patients will
have acute tubular necrosis (ATN). ATN is an acute,
potentially reversible decrease in renal function resulting from toxic or ischemic injury to the kidneys.[7]
Mazze, in a review of a large number of cases of ATN
in several centers, found that 43 per cent of cases of
acute renal failure were related to surgery and 9 per
cent to trauma.[8]

**TABLE 11–6. Causes of Acute Renal Failure**

**Prerenal—Inadequate Perfusion**
Intravascular volume depletion (any cause)
Cardiac failure
Hypotension
Vascular obstruction

**Intrinsic Renal—Inadequate Organ Function**
Acute tubular necrosis
  Ischemic
  Nephrotoxicities

Medical causes
  Vasculitis
  Malignant hypertension
  Tubular obstruction
  Hepatorenal
  Hypercalcemia
  Sepsis

**Postrenal—Inadequate Drainage**
Bladder outlet obstruction
  Enlarged prostate or hypotonic bladder
  Carcinoma
  Obstructed drainage device

Ureteral obstruction
  Accidental ligature
  Extrinsic compression secondary to hematoma or carcinoma
  Stones, clots, papillary tissues

The two basic mechanisms of acute tubular necrosis are ischemic and nephrotoxic insults.

(1) Ischemic insults: Ischemic insults are caused by reduced blood flow to the kidneys.[9, 10] In most surgical cases these factors include preoperative fluid depletion, the effect of the anesthesia, and interoperative fluid loss. Although most patients tolerate the insult of the surgery and anesthesia, complicating factors, such as previous hypertension, nephrotoxins, dehydration, or sepsis, may magnify the insult, resulting in acute renal failure (see Table 11–7).

Because ischemic renal injury is one of the major causes of ATN, every effort should be made to bring the patient to the operating room in an optimum state of hydration to prevent this complication.

(2) Nephrotoxins: Nephrotoxic injury is the second

### TABLE 11–7. Causes of Ischemia

Volume depletion owing to blood loss, inadequate IV therapy, "third space" sequestration, excessive G.I. or renal losses
Severe vasoconstriction as with pressor agents or cardiac failure
Hypotension
Cardiac failure
Obstructive jaundice*
Interruption of flow, cross-damping aorta, or embolus†
Liver failure
Nephrotic syndrome
Sepsis

*Patients with obstructive jaundice are prone to develop acute renal failure with and without surgery. The exact relationship between the jaundice and renal failure is not clear. (In patients with markedly elevated bilirubin, an infusion of 10% mannitol for diuresis is recommended, beginning two hours before surgery, to maintain a urinary output of 50 to 100 ml/hour for 48 hours postoperatively. Appropriate caution should avoid dehydration or hypokalemia.[11, 12, 13, 14, 15])

†Surgery of abdominal aortic aneurysm is frequently associated with acute renal failure. The ischemic mechanism is likely that of ischemia from cross-clamping the aorta above the level of the renal arteries. Although the "safe" period of cross-clamping is said to be 30 minutes in normal patients, it is considerably shorter in patients with preexisting renal disease. Some authors recommend a mannitol infusion before and immediately after surgery in an effort to prevent acute renal failure.

most common cause of ATN. A partial list of nephrotoxins include the antibiotics (aminoglycosides, polymyxins, and rifampin), heme pigments (hemoglobin), the heavy metals (mercury, arsenic, and platinum); radiocontrast materials, carbon tetrachloride, methoxyflurane, and acetazolamide.

(a) Aminoglycosides: Of the nephrotoxins, gentamicin is the most common agent to cause recognized renal failure.[16] Gentamicin toxicity is enhanced by volume depletion, underlying renal disease, and age. Increased gentamicin serum levels, as well as the simultaneous administration of cephalothin, also increase the renal toxicity.

(b) Radiocontrast agents: Iodinated radiocontrast agents cause acute renal failure and should be used judiciously, particularly in those patients who have underlying renal risk factors. Alternative imaging with nuclear scans or ultrasonography is safer. When radiocontrast materials must be used, adequate hydration is essential.[17]

Intravenous pyelography is dangerous in diabetic patients, especially those with elevated serum creatinines.[18, 19] Harkonen noted 76 per cent incidence of acute renal injury after intravenous pyelography with serum creatinine of over 2 mg/dl. VanZee and co-workers found that when the serum creatinine was more than 4.5 mg/dl, 31 per cent of hypertension patients and 100 per cent of diabetic patients developed acute renal injury.[19]

(c) Heme pigments: Both hemoglobin and myoglobin are nephrotoxins. Myoglobinuria from tissue destruction may be present in those patients with extensive burns or trauma or those undergoing surgery on ischemic limbs. Rhabdomyolysis with release of myoglobin may also occur from seizures, alcoholism, and other metabolic derangements.[20]

Intravascular hemolysis from transfusion mismatch or cardiopulmonary bypass produces hemoglobinuria.

Dehydration potentiates nephrotoxicity from heme pigments and from any other cause.

c. Postrenal acute renal failure: Postrenal causes are obstruction anywhere from the renal pelvis to the urethra that prevents excretion of urine. Because obstruction is potentially reversible, it is important to consider this a cause of acute renal failure. Typically, the urine volume is less than 200 ml. In the male patient with prostatic obstruction, the bladder may be distended.

2. Prerenal versus intrinsic renal disease: In the presence of oliguric renal failure and the absence of bladder distention or anuria, the differential diagnosis is between prerenal and renal oliguria.

In the prerenal state the kidney is maximally reabsorbing salt and water to compensate for hypoperfusion. Consequently, the urinalysis will show specific gravity greater than 1.015, osmolarity greater than 350 mOsm/L, urinary sodium less than 10 mEq/L, and normal urinary sediment. There may be clinical evidence of dehydration.

On the other hand, those patients with renal azotemia (ATN) have urine specific gravity less than 1.015 and urine sodium greater than 20 mEq/L. There may be

TABLE 11–8. Findings in Prerenal Azotemia and Acute Tubular Necrosis*

|  | Prerenal Azotemia | Acute Tubular Necrosis |
|---|---|---|
| Urine sodium | < 10 mEq/L | > 20–25 mEq/L |
| Urine specific gravity | > 1.015 | < 1.010–1.015 |
| Urine sediment | Normal | Broad brown casts Cellular debris |
| Intavascular volume depletion | Yes | Variable |
| Spun microscopic urine | Waxy cast | Dirty brown cellular casts |

*Previous diuretic therapy make these values difficult to interpret.

polyuria and abnormal urinary sediment with casts and red or white cells. Clinically, the patient may be euhydrated, dehydrated or overhydrated. Those patients who are dehydrated should be rehydrated and reassessed. Table 11–8 summarizes these findings.

If prerenal azotemia is suspected, begin hydration before laboratory values are available.

3. Perioperative management

   a. Management of the oliguric patient with prerenal azotemia: When the diagnosis of prerenal azotemia is made, intravascular volume is rapidly repleted with intravenous fluids. The results of the infusion will be of both diagnostic and therapeutic value, as the introduction of several hundred milliliters of saline to the dehydrated patient should result in increased urinary output. When oliguria persists despite fluid therapy, the possibilities are that (1) the original diagnosis of prerenal azotemia was in error; (2) the fluid challenge was insufficient to correct the prerenal cause; (3) treatment was not instituted promptly enough to prevent postischemic ATN.

   In those patients wtih cardiac or pulmonary disease, it may be necessary to insert a Swan-Ganz catheter to measure pulmonary wedge pressures.

   Although controversial, some recommend that 200 to 400 mg of furosemide be given IV in an effort to convert oliguric renal failure to nonoliguric renal failure with improvement in prognosis.

b. Management of acute tubular necrosis: Management of acute tubular necrosis, as with other types of acute renal failure, is directed at maintaining the balance of fluid, electrolytes, and pH. Hyponatremia and hyperkalemia are the most common electrolyte disturbances. The main indication for dialysis are hyperkemia, fluid overload, hyponatremia, severe acidosis, and uremic complications. The role for prophylactic dialysis is unclear. However, in patients with severe trauma or extreme catabolic states, early dialysis may be indicated.[21]

Maintenance of nutrition is extremely important in patients with acute renal failure. This should be accomplished orally, when possible. Hyperalimentation is available if needed.[22]

## REFERENCES

1. Hata M, Remmers AR, Lindley JD, et al: Surgical management of the dialysis patient. Ann Surg *178*:134, 1973.
2. Brenowitz JB, Williams CD, Edwards WS: Major surgery in patients with chronic renal failure. Am J Surg *134*:765, 1977.
3. Herrin JT: Preparation of the renal patient for surgery. Int Anesthesiol Clin *13*:183, 1975.
4. Haimov M, Glabman S, Shupak E, et al: General surgery in patients on maintenance hemodialysis. Ann Surg *179*:863, 1974.
5. Stuart FP, Simowian SJ, Hill JL: Special considerations in surgical management of patients on hemodialysis and after successful kidney transplantation. Surg Clin North Am *56*:15, 1976.
6. Bennett WM, Singer I, Golper T, et al: Guidelines for drug therapy in renal failure. Ann Intern Med *86*:754, 1977.
7. Grossman RA: Oliguria and acute renal failure. Med Clin North Am *65*:419, 1981.
8. Mazze I: Critical care of the patient with acute renal failure. Anesthesiology *17*:138, 1977.
9. Balslov JT, Jorgensen HE: A survey of 499 patients with acute anuric renal insufficiency: Causes, treatment, complications, and mortality. Am J Med *34*:753, 1963.
10. Deutsch S: Effects of anesthetics on the kidney. Surg Clin North Am *55*:775, 1975.
11. Dawson JL: Jaundice and anoxic renal damage: Protective effect of mannitol. Br Med J *1*:810, 1964.
12. Dawson JL: Post-operative renal function in obstructive jaundice: Effect of mannitol diuresis. Br Med J *1*:82, 1965.
13. Sorenson FH, Anderson JB, Ornsholt J, Skjoldborg H: Acute renal failure complicating biliary tract disorders. Acta Chir Scand *137*:87, 1971.

14. Williams RD, Elliot DW, Zollinger RM: The effect of hypotension in obstructive jaundice. Arch Surg *81*:344, 1960.

15. Bloom D, McCalden TA, Rosendorff C: Effects of jaundiced plasma on vascular sensitivity to noradrenalin. Kidney Int *8*:149, 1975.

16. Appel GB, Neu HC: Nephrotoxicity of antimicrobial agents. N Engl J Med *296*:663, 772, 784, 1977.

17. Pendergross EP, Hodes JP, Tondreau RL, et al: Further consideration of deaths and unfavorable sequelae following administration of contrast media and angiography in the United States. Am J Roentgenol *74*:228, 1955.

18. Harkonen S, Kjellstrand CM: Exacerbation of diabetic renal failure following mitrovenous pyelography. Am J Med *63*:939, 1977.

19. VanZee BE, Hoy WE, Talley TE, Jaenike JR: Renal injury associated with intravenous pyelography in nondiabetic and diabetic patients. Ann Intern Med *89*:51, 1978.

20. Jaenike JR: Micropuncture study of methemoglobin-induced acute renal failure. J Lab Clin Med *73*:459, 1969.

21. Conger JD: A controlled evaluation of prophylactic dialysis in acute renal failure. J Trauma *15*:1056, 1975.

22. Abel RM, Beck C, Abbott WN, et al: Improved survival from acute renal failure after treatment with intravenous essential L-amino acids and glucose. N Engl J Med *288*:695, 1973.

# 12

# THE NERVOUS SYSTEM

Preoperative evaluation and management of patients with neurologic disease requires an understanding of the specific disease entities. Because neurologic disorders are unique in their pathophysiology and in their relationship to anesthesia, those most commonly encountered will be discussed individually. Operative risk is often related to neuromuscular impairment of pulmonary function or cardiac function, and thus any numerical risk analysis related to the disease itself is difficult to assess. Therefore, an awareness of the peculiarities of each disease and which factors can be modified to reduce risk is the key to good perioperative management.

## I. MYASTHENIA GRAVIS

### A. PREOPERATIVE EVALUATION

1. Background and purpose

    Myasthenia gravis is an autoimmune disease. It is characterized by remitting and relapsing muscle weakness and fatigability resulting from a defect in neuromuscular transmission. Its etiology is believed to involve antiacetylcholine antibodies that bind to the nicotinic acetylcholine receptors. The antibodies are of the IgG class. Management techniques have changed recently, with early thymectomy, anticholinesterases, steroids, immunosuppression, and plasmapheresis taking their place in the armamentarium of treatment. When the internist is called for preoperative evaluation of a patient with myasthenia gravis, knowledge of such therapies is important.

2. Clinical assessment

    a. History

      (1) Documentation of past thymectomy or other

surgeries and any complications associated with them
(2) Medications
b. Physical examination
(1) Attention to pulmonary ausculation and percussion. Evaluation of pulmonary function and muscle debility is particularly important.
c. Laboratory studies
(1) CBC and platelets
(2) Prothrombin time and thromboplastin time
(3) Electrolytes, BUN, and glucose
(4) Pulmonary function tests
(5) Arterial blood gas
(6) Chest x-ray
(7) ECG

## B. PERIOPERATIVE MANAGEMENT

1. Premedication should be kept at a minimum—especially respiratory depressants.
2. Local anesthetics of the ester group (cocaine, procaine, amethocaine) are hydrolyzed by cholinesterase and should be avoided.
3. Local anesthetics of the amide group (lidocaine, prilocaine, mepivacaine, bupivacaine), which are metabolized in the liver, should be used.
4. On the day before surgery, anticholinesterases are stopped after the last daily dose. This will influence favorably the acetylcholine-insensitive state and decrease the resistance of the patient to anticholinesterases postoperatively.
5. Postoperatively, IM or parenteral anticholinesterases (pyridostigmine or neostigmine) are administered at one thirtieth the oral dose every four to six hours. Oral medications are restarted when the patient is able to take medications by mouth.
6. Table 12–1 lists the various anticholinesterases used in the treatment of myasthenia gravis and their equivalent doses.
7. Postoperatively, particular attention should be given to pulmonary care. Initial postoperative care in the ICU is recommended after general anesthesia. Deep breathing, incentive spirometry, postural drainage, and percussion are emphasized in the postoperative period.

**TABLE 12–1. Therapeutic Regimen for Myasthenia Gravis**

| Drug | Dose | Frequency |
| --- | --- | --- |
| Pyridostigmine (Mestinon) | PO, 60 mg<br>Liquid 5 ml =<br>60 mg<br>IM, IV* | q4–6h |
| Neostigmine (Prostigmin) | PO, 15 mg<br>IM, IV* | q4–6h |
| Ambenonium (Mytelase) | PO, 30 mg | q4–6h |

*Parenteral dose is one thirtieth of total oral dose.

## C. SPECIAL CONSIDERATIONS

1. Thymectomy

    Thymectomy has been advocated to improve patients clinically and may possibly result in remission of the disease. This area is controversial, however. With the present modern management, the operative mortality is 0.6 per cent.[1] Only 10 per cent of patients with myasthenia gravis will have thymoma.[2, 3]

2. Anticholinesterases

    Pyridostigmine is the most commonly used drug in myasthenia gravis. The results of a study done by Cohan and co-workers show the gastrointestinal absorption of this drug to be poor and that its peak action is approximately two hours after ingestion.[4] Duration of action is between four and a half and six hours.[2] Somani and associates[5] identified a metabolite of pyridostigmine in myasthenic patients that may accumulate and contribute to overdosage problems.

3. Steroids

    When high-dose prednisone therapy (50 to 100 mg) is initiated in myasthenia gravis, approximately 8 per cent of patients will have exacerbation of myasthenia weakness.[6] This is ascribed to an interaction of corticosteroid with the anticholinesterase drugs (pyridostigmine).[6] Seybold and Drachman have recommended beginning steroid therapy with low doses and then increasing the dose gradually to minimize this weakness.[7] Anticholinesterase drugs must be readjusted during therapy with corticosteroid to optimize response.

4. Immunosuppression

   Azathioprine or 6-mercaptopurine has proved helpful in 80 per cent to 89 per cent of cases, often after unsuccessful treatment with prednisone and thymectomy.[8, 9]

5. Plasmapheresis

   Plasmapheresis is now being used in patients with severe or progressive myasthenia gravis who have not responded to other therapy.[10] Its function is to remove circulating acetylcholine reception antibodies. Newsom-Davis and associates did not demonstrate any difference in clinical response between immunosuppression plus plasmapheresis and immunosuppressive drugs alone.[11, 12] Although complications are uncommon, plasmapheresis can cause electrolyte imbalance, severe muscle cramps, thrombosis, and removal of clotting factors and plasma-bound drugs.

## REFERENCES

1. Cohen HE, Solit RW, Shatz NJ, et al: Surgical treatment in myasthenia gravis in 27 years experience. J Thorac Cardiovasc Surg 68:876, 1974.
2. Patten BE: Myasthenia gravis: Review of diagnosis and management. Muscle Nerve 1:190, 1978.
3. Castleman B: The pathology of the thymus gland in myasthenia gravis. Ann NY Acad Sci 135:496, 1963.
4. Cohan SL, Pahlmann LW, Mitszewski J, O'Doherty DS: The pharmacokinetics of pyridostigmine. Neurology 26:536, 1976.
5. Somani SM, Roberts JB, Wilson A: Pyridostigmine metabolism in man. Clin Pharmacol Ther 13:393, 1972.
6. Pahen BM, Oliver KL, Engle WK: Adverse interaction between steroid hormones and anticholinesterase drugs. Neurology 24:442, 1974.
7. Seybold ME, Drachman DB: Gradually increasing doses of prednisone in myasthenia gravis: Reducing the hazard of treatment. N Engl J Med 290:81, 1974.
8. Matell G, Bergstrom K, Franksson C, et al: Effects of some immunosuppressive procedures on myasthenia gravis. Ann NY Acad Sci 274:659, 1976.
9. Mertens HG, Balzereit F, Leipert M: The treatment of severe myasthenia gravis with immunosuppressive agents. Eur Neurol 2:321, 1969.
10. Dau PC, Lindstrom JM, Cassell CK, et al: Plasmapheresis and immunosuppressive drug therapy in myasthenia gravis. N Engl J Med 297:1134, 1977.
11. Newsom-Davis J, Pinching AJ, Vincent A, et al: Function of

circulating antibody to acetylcholine receptor in myasthenia gravis: Investigation by plasma exchange. Neurology *28*:266, 1978.

12. Newsom-Davis J, Wilson SG, Vincent A, et al: Long term effects of repeated plasma exchange in myasthenia gravis. Lancet *1*:464, 1979.

## II. SEIZURE DISORDER

### A. PREOPERATIVE EVALUATION

1. Background and purpose

   The statistics of Hauser and Kurland[1] show that at least one million persons in the United States are subject to recurrent seizures and that at least ten times that number consult a physician or go to a hospital some time in their lives because of a seizure. Seizures are the sudden onset of a disorderly discharge of neurons from a normal or diseased cerebral cortex. There are four categories of seizures: (1) generalized tonic-clonic (grand mal), (2) complex partial (temporal lobe, psychomotor), (3) simple partial (focal), and (4) absence (petit mal). The preoperative consultant assessing a patient with a known seizure disorder must consider a history of seizure recurrence and the adequacy of the medication regimen used. Evans[2] reported that various anesthetic agents can lower seizure thresholds, produce high-frequency EEG activity, and precipitate seizures. Therefore, appropriate preoperative assessment of seizure history, drug compliance, and serum levels of seizure medication are important to best prepare the patient for anesthesia.

2. Clinical assessment

   a. History of frequency of seizures, precipitating etiologies (e.g., alcohol), and medication history should be obtained.

   b. Patients with seizure disorders necessitating surgery can be classified as shown in Table 12–2.

   c. Laboratory studies
      (1) CBC
      (2) Electrolytes, BUN, glucose
      (3) Chest x-ray
      (4) ECG
      (5) Levels of antiepileptic drugs

TABLE 12–2. Classification of Seizure Disorder and Type of Surgery Permitted

| Classification | Permissible Surgery |
|---|---|
| Known, well controlled | Elective surgery |
| Known, poorly controlled | Elective surgery |
| Known only | Emergency surgery |

Adapted from Garvin JS: Management of convulsions in surgical patients. Surg Annu *11*:25, 1971.

## B. PERIOPERATIVE MANAGEMENT

1. Average loading and maintenance doses plus the therapeutic levels for phenytoin and phenobarbital are listed in Table 12–3. (Loading doses are for previously untreated patients.)
2. The phenytoin oral loading dose schedule by Wilder and associates[3] can be used in patients not currently treated:

    400 mg + 300 mg + 300 mg = 1000 mg
    (give at two-hour intervals)

3. The following formula[4] is used to calculate the loading dose necessary to elevate the known subtherapeutic level of phenytoin or phenobarbital into therapeutic range in patients suboptimally treated:

$$\text{Loading dose} = \frac{V (C_D - C_o)}{F}$$

V = volume of distribution (0.65 L/kg for phenytoin and 0.60 L/kg for phenobarbital

TABLE 12–3. Phenytoin and Phenobarbital Dosages

Phenytoin
  Loading dose: 15–18 mg/kg
  Maintenance: 4–8 mg/kg/day
  Therapeutic: 10–20 μg/ml

Phenobarbital
  Loading dose: 2–6 mg/kg
  Maintenance: 1–5 mg/kg/day
  Therapeutic: 15–40 μg/ml

$C_D$ = concentration of phenytoin or phenobarbital desired

$C_o$ = concentration of phenytoin or phenobarbital observed

$F$ = bioavailability IV = 1.0
$$PO = 0.95 \text{ phenytoin}$$
$$0.90 \text{ phenobarbital}$$

    4. Phenytoin and phenobarbital schedules based on the classification in Table 12–2 are shown in Table 12–4.

**TABLE 12–4. Phenytoin and Phenobarbital Schedules**

|  |  |  |
|---|---|---|
| | **Known, well controlled — elective surgery** | |
| Schedule A | Phenytoin | Day before: Regular dose |
| | | Postop: Resume PO |
| | Phenobarbital | Postop/NPO: IV or IM* |
| | **Known, poorly controlled — elective surgery** | |
| Schedule B | (Drug level zero) | Day before: Load IV or PO |
| | Phenytoin | Postop: Resume PO |
| | Phenobarbital | Postop/NPO: IV or IM* |
| | (Drug level subtherapeutic)† | Day before: Load IV, IM,* or PO |
| | Phenytoin | Postop: Resume PO |
| | Phenobarbital | Postop/NPO: IV or IM* |
| | **Known — emergency surgery** | |
| Schedule C | Assess history and categorize patient. | |
| | Apply Schedule A and B. | |

*Phenobarbital only
†Formula above

5. The pharmacologic properties of six antiepileptic drugs are shown in Table 12–5.
6. Phenytoin is the most frequently used seizure medication, and the following points should always be kept in mind:
   a. Phenytoin should be used only in saline solution of lactated Ringer's.
   b. IM phenytoin will precipitate at the injection site, and absorption is erratic. We refrain from using it in this manner.
   c. Cardiovascular collapse and central nervous system depression are the major toxicities observed on IV administration, and the rate should never exceed 50 mg/min. This reaction is due primarily to the propylene glycol diluent.

## C. SPECIAL CONSIDERATIONS

1. Head trauma
2. Brain tumors
3. Craniotomy

The recommendation from the neurosurgery literature is to give the patient with these problems phenytoin. (See Table 12–3 for recommended phenytoin doses.)

## REFERENCES

1. Hauser WA, Kurland LT: The epidemiology of epilepsy in Rochester, Minnesota. Epilepsia *16*:1, 1975.
2. Evans DE: Anaesthesia and the epileptic patient: A review. Anaesthesia *30*:34–45, 1975.
3. Wilder BS, Romsay RE, Willmore LJ, Fenstein GF, Perchalski RS, Shumale JB: Efficacy of intravenous phenytoin in the treatment of suspected epileptics: Kinetics of CNS penetration. Ann Neurol *1*:511–518, 1977.
4. Tozer TN, Winter ME: Phenytoin, in Evans WE, Schentag JJ, Jusko WJ (eds): Applied Pharmacokinetics. San Francisco, Applied Therapeutics, 1980, p 296.

## III. PARKINSONISM

### A. PREOPERATIVE EVALUATION

1. Background and purpose
   Parkinsonism is the most common of the disorders of the extrapyramidal system and the most prevalent of the primary disorders of the central nervous system. Parkinsonism presents with these cardinal signs: resting tremor,

**TABLE 12–5. Pharmacologic Properties of Six Antiepileptic Drugs**

| Drug | Dosage (mg/day) | Expected Blood Level | | Time to Reach Steady-State Blood Levels (days) | Serum Half-Life (h) | Effective Blood Level (μg/ml) | Toxic Blood Level (μg/ml) | Protein Bound (%) |
| | | Average (μg/ml) | Range (μg/ml) | | | | | |
| --- | --- | --- | --- | --- | --- | --- | --- | --- |
| Phenytoin (Dilantin) | 300 | 10 | 5–20 | 5–10 | $24 \pm 12$ | >10 | >20 | 90 |
| Phenobarbital (Luminal) | 120 | 20 | 10–30 | 14–21 | $96 \pm 12$ | >15 | >40 | 40–50 |
| Primidone (Mysoline) | 750 | 8 | 5–15 | 4–7 | $12 \pm 6$ | >5 | >12 | 0–50 |
| Phenobarbital | Derived | 24 | 5–32 | 14–21 | — | — | — | — |
| Carbamazepine (Tegretol) | 1200 | 6 | 3–12 | 2–4 | $12 \pm 3$ | >4 | >8 | 70 |
| Valproic acid (Depakene) | 1500 | 50 | 40–70 | 2–4 | $12 \pm 6$ | >50 | >100 | 90 |
| Ethosuximide (Zarontin) | 1000 | 60 | 40–100 | 5–8 | $30 \pm 6$ | >40 | >100 | 0 |

From Penry JK, Newmark ME: The use of antiepileptic drugs. Ann Intern Med 90:207–218, 1979. Reproduced with permission.

ridigity, and hypokinesia. Parkinsonism can be classified into three groups based on etiology: primary or idiopathic, secondary or symptomatic (infection or drug), and paraparkinsonian disorder (Shy-Drager syndrome, Wilson's disease). Of major concern in preoperative evaluation are the proper use of antiparkinsonism drugs and the complications they may provoke.

2. Clinical assessment

   a. Cardiac: Goldberg[1] has reported that the most significant complication of levodopa therapy is the effect of dopamine on the cardiovascular system. The drug stimulates myocardial beta-adrenergic receptors that, in the presence of myocardial ischemia or a sensitizing anesthetic agent (cyclopropane or halothane), could cause cardiac dysrhythmias. Hypotension is another side affect of levodopa, levodopa-carbidopa, and bromocriptine and must be monitored for postoperatively. MacIntyre and co-workers[2] and Bevan and co-workers[3] have reported two cases of postoperative hypotension in patients with parkinsonism treated with levodopa. No increased incidence of operative complications was reported.

   b. Pulmonary: Paulson and Tafrate[4] have reported that ventilatory insufficiency secondary to increased chest wall rigidity and salivation from difficulty in swallowing could become postoperative problems in Parkinson's disease. Pulmonary function testing is frequently indicated.

### TABLE 12–6. Drugs with Dopaminergic Action

| Drug | Dose | Action |
|------|------|--------|
| Levodopa (Dopar, Larodopa) | 1 tab, PO, t.i.d. or q.i.d. (100 mg, 250 mg, 500 mg) | Dopamine availability |
| Levodopa-carbidopa (Sinemet) | 1 tab, PO, t.i.d. or q.i.d. (10/100, 25/100, 25/250) | |
| Bromocriptine (Parlodel) | 1 tab, PO, b.i.d. (2.5 mg, 5 mg) | Activates dopaminergic receptors |
| Amantadine (Symmetrel) | 100 mg, PO, b.i.d. | Increases dopamine release |
| Carbidopa | (see levodopa-carbidopa) | Dopamine metabolism |

**TABLE 12–7. Drugs with Cholinergic Action**

| Drug | Dose | Action |
|------|------|--------|
| Cycrimine (Pagitane) | 1.2–5 mg PO t.i.d. | Block cholinergic receptors |
| Procyclidine (Kemadrin) | 2–2.5 mg PO t.i.d. | |
| Trihexyphenidyl (Artane) | 6–10 mg PO q.i.d. (divided doses) | |
| Benztropine (Cogentin) | 0.5–6 mg PO b.i.d. | |
| Biperiden (Akineton) | 2 mg PO t.i.d. | |
| Diphenhydramine (Benedryl) | | Antihistamine anticholinergics |
| Chlorphenoxamine (Phenoxene) | Rarely used | |
| Orphenadrine (Disipal) | | |

## B. PERIOPERATIVE MANAGEMENT

1. Antiparkinsonism agents (Tables 12–6 and 12–7)
2. Levodopa has a short half-life and must be given every six hours. If the therapy is stopped the night before surgery, little dopamine will be present in the peripheral adrenergic tissue.[5] If the patient remains NPO for some time, restart the medication at lower doses and gradually increase to preoperative doses to avoid side effects.
3. If the patient is taking anticholinergic agents, atropine should be eliminated as a preoperative medication, since its action is similar to these agents.
4. Bromocriptine has a long half-life and is administered every 12 hours.[6, 7] Hypotension can occur and is believed to be due to a relaxation of vascular smooth muscle in the splanchnic and renal circulation, inhibition of transmitter release at noradrenergic nerve endings, and central inhibition of sympathetic activity.[7, 8]

## REFERENCES

1. Goldberg LI: Levodopa and anesthesia. Anesthesiology *34*:1, 1971.
2. MacIntyre IM, Strange DM, Beavis JP: L-Dopa and general anesthesia. Anesthesiology *26*:370, 1971.
3. Bevan DR, Monks PS, Calne DB: Cardiovascular reactions to anesthesia during treatment with levadopa. Anesthesiology *28*:29, 1973.
4. Paulson CD, Tafrate RH: Some "minor" aspects of parkinsonism, especially pulmonary function. Neurology *20*(suppl):14–17, 1970.

5. Ngai SH: Parkinsonism, levodopa, and anesthesia. Anesthesiology *37*:344, 1972.

6. Parkes D: Bromocriptine. N Engl J Med *301*:873, 1979.

7. Clark BJ, Scholtyski C, Fluckiger E: Cardiovascular actions of bromocriptine. Acta Endocrinol *216*(suppl):75–81, 1978.

8. Quinn N, Illas A, Lhermihe F, Agid I: Bromocriptine in Parkinson's disease: A study of cardiovascular effects. J Neurol Neurosurg Pyschiatry *44*:426–428, 1981.

## IV. MUSCULAR DYSTROPHY

### A. PREOPERATIVE EVALUATION

1. Background and purpose

   Muscular dystrophy can be divided into four main groups: (1) Duchenne's, (2) Becker's pseudohypertrophic (Duchenne's) muscular dystrophy, (3) facioscapulohumeral syndrome, (4) myotonic dystrophy (a sex-linked recessive disorder commonly seen in males before age six). It is a progressive degenerative disease. Becker's dystrophy is a sex-linked recessive disorder similar to Duchenne's dystrophy but pursues a milder course and has a better prognosis. The facioscapulohumeral syndrome is an autosomal dominant disorder with complete penetrance that is seen equally in males and females in the second and third decades. Myotonic dystrophy is an autosomal dominant disorder that appears most commonly in males after the third decade. This disorder is the type of muscular dystrophy encountered most frequently in a general hospital. It is a distal myopathy, unlike the other dystrophies, which are proximal. When assessing these patients preoperatively, cardiac, pulmonary, and endocrine factors should be evaluated.

2. Clinical assessment

   a. Cardiac:[1, 2] Duchenne's and myotonic dystrophy are more commonly associated with cardiac problems, ranging from tachycardia, bradycardia, conduction defects, and extrasystoles to cardiac arrest. The estimated frequency of ECG abnormalities accompanying myotonic dystrophy is between 85 per cent and 90 per cent. The most common of these abnormalities are prolonged PR and QRS intervals. Atrial arrhythmias are more common than ventricular arrhythmias. Complete heart block occurs infrequently but should be watched for in these patients. Cardiac monitoring is essential.

    b. Pulmonary:[3, 4] As the disease progresses, respiratory muscle involvement results in a restrictive pattern with the inability to clear secretions. Pulmonary function tests and arterial blood gases should be obtained when indicated.

    c. Endocrine:[3, 4] Patients with myotonic dystrophy may manifest diabetes mellitus, hypothyroidism, and androgen deficiencies. Blood sugar and thyroid studies are important.

## B. PERIOPERATIVE MANAGEMENT

1. A temporary pacemaker is placed when the following conditions are present: symptomatic bifascicular block, complete heart block; Mobitz II second degree block with or without symptoms.
2. Phenytoin 100 mg PO t.i.d. is the treatment of choice for myotonic dystrophy if episodes of myotonia affect normal life functions.[5]
3. Recommended postoperative pulmonary care includes incentive spirometry, deep breathing, postural drainage, and percussion.

## *REFERENCES*

1. Dewind LT, Jones RJ: Cardiovascular observations in dystrophia myotonia. JAMA *144*:299, 1950.
2. Moha J, Guilleminault C, Billingham M, Barry W, Mason J: Cardiac abnormalities in myotonic dystrophy. Am J Med *67*:467, 1979.
3. Cobham IG, Davis HS: Anesthesia for muscular dystrophy patients. Anesth Analg *43*:22, 1964.
4. Kaufman L: Anesthesia in dystrophia myotonia. Proc Roy Soc Med *53*:183, 1959.
5. Griggs RC, Davies RJ, Anderson DC, et al: Cardiac conduction in myotonic dystrophy. Am J Med *59*:37, 1975.

# 13

# SPECIAL CONSIDERATIONS

## I. THE HEALTHY PATIENT

### A. PREOPERATIVE EVALUATION

1. Purpose
   a. To determine the appropriate preoperative workup in surgical patients who are considered healthy. Healthy patients are defined by the American Society of Anesthesiologists as Class I physical status: "No disease other than surgical pathology, no systemic disturbances."[1]
   b. Risk factors
      (1) Family history (e.g., anemia, bleeding disorders, hypertension, diabetes mellitus, coronary artery disease)
      (2) Smoking
      (3) Drug allergies
      (4) Alcohol intake
2. Clinical assessment
   To evaluate a patient for surgery properly, several questions must be asked: (1) What type of surgery is contemplated and what are its risks? (2) What type of anesthesia will be used and what are its risks? (3) What inherent risk factors does the patient have?

Detailed analysis of the first two questions is beyond the scope of this manual, but the following can be said. Those patients who fit the definition of a healthy patient usually are younger than forty-five. The most common operative procedures performed on the employees of the Metropolitan Life Insurance Company in the age-group twenty-five to forty-five are shown in Table 13–1. Most of the procedures were elective and the mortality was low. Because the mortality is low it is important to evaluate these patients properly to ensure there is no underlying disease process that will add to the surgical mortality.

TABLE 13–1. Annual Number of Surgical Procedures and Death Rate per 1000 Population

| Surgical Procedures | HEW (Age 15–44) | Metropolitan Life (Age 25–45) | Death Rate |
|---|---|---|---|
| Dilatation and curettage | 8.86 | 1.090 | 0.10 |
| Hysterectomy | 4.77 | 7.00 | 0.25 |
| Bilateral tubal ligation | 3.97 | | 0.04 |
| Ovariectomy | 2.77 | 1.10 | 0.30 |
| Tonsillectomy | 2.28 | 1.00 | 0.06 |
| Appendectomy | 1.93 | 1.00 | 0.13 |
| Cholecystectomy | 1.84 | 1.15 | 0.30 |
| Inguinal hernia repair | 1.46 | 2.50* | 0.11 |

*Males only
From Robbins JA, Mushlin AI: Preoperative evaluation of the healthy patient. Med Clin North Am *63*:1145–1156, 1979.

a. History: The preoperative history should be similar to that taken for other reasons except that emphasis should be placed on finding medical problems that may have some bearing on the outcome of surgery. Some of these problems are listed in Table 13–2.

In addition to the conditions listed in Table 13–2 several other points must be considered:

(1) Has the patient had surgery before? If so, were there any complications, anesthesia-related or otherwise?

(2) If the patient is a premenopausal female, is there a possibility of pregnancy?

(3) Is there a history of drug allergy?

(4) Does the patient smoke? How much?

(5) Is there a history of significant alcohol intake?

TABLE 13–2. Medical Conditions That May Have a Detrimenal Effect on Surgical Outcome

| | |
|---|---|
| Anemia | Cardiac valvular disease |
| Bleeding disorders | Cardiac arrhythmias |
| Thrombocytopenia | Liver disease |
| Diabetes mellitus | Renal disease |
| Coronary artery disorder | Chronic obstructive pulmonary disease |

    b. Physical examination: The physical examination should focus on finding asymptomatic disease processes that might affect surgical outcome.

        (1) Vital signs should be measured, with close attention to the blood pressure to rule out undiagnosed hypertension.

        (2) The skin should be examined for signs of anemia (pallor) or bleeding disorders (petechiae, bruising). Signs of liver disease may also be present (jaundice, spider angiomata, palmar erythema).

        (3) Ocular examination may point to anemia (pale conjunctiva) or liver disease (scleral icterus). Fundoscopic examination may show changes consistent with diabetes mellitus or hypertension.

        (4) On oral examination, look for impediments to easy endotracheal intubation.

        (5) Neck examination should include auscultation of the carotid arteries for possible stenotic lesions.

        (6) Pulmonary examination may reveal signs of chronic obstructive pulmonary disease (decreased breath sounds, wheezing or rales), which may indicate early heart failure or pneumonia.

        (7) Cardiovascular system examination should include careful auscultation of the heart for valvular murmurs, especially mitral valve prolapse. Major arteries should be auscultated for bruits. Rhythm should be assessed.

        (8) Careful palpation of the abdomen should be performed to rule out hepatosplenomegaly or aortic aneurysm.

        (9) Rectal examination should include testing the stool for occult blood.

     (10) Close inspection of the legs should be done to detect venous varicosities, which are a major risk factor for development of deep venous thrombosis.

    c. Laboratory assessment: If during the history or physical examination evidence for another disorder is found, surgery should be canceled if at all possible and a workup begun. Assuming no other abnormalities are found, what further laboratory testing should be done?

        Various studies have been made of the usefulness of several tests for screening purposes. Robbins and Rose[2] looked at the partial thromboplastin time (PTT) and in their retrospective analysis of 1025 PTT measurements found 43 abnormal results. All the patients who had abnormal results also had some indication, by history or physical examination, of the disorder.

In like manner, Bonebrake and associates[3] looked at the practical value of the routine chest x-ray in pregnant patients. They retrospectively reviewed the records of 12,109 consecutive deliveries at the Mayo Clinic and found 48 abnormal chest x-rays. Once again, in every case the abnormality could have been predicted from the history or physical examination.

Robbins and Mushlin[4] have attempted to consolidate material from many sources and to generate a reasonable approach to the healthy patient. They have outlined five criteria to help determine whether or not a test is helpful as a preoperative screen.

(1) The condition must be asymptomatic and not obvious on physical examination or by history.

(2) The condition must affect the patient's morbidity and mortality or possibly affect those who are involved in the patient's care.

(3) Preoperative diagnosis must be more beneficial to the patient's management than diagnosis in the intra- or postoperative period.

(4) The test available must be both sensitive and specific to make the diagnosis.

(5) The condition must be common enough so that an abnormal result most likely indicates disease.

Goldman[5] added a sixth criterion, which is that the surgical admission provides an excellent opportunity to do appropriate testing recommended for periodic screening of the healthy patient.

Robbins and Mushlin[4] also developed two interesting tables. The first (Table 13–3) outlined the sensitivity and specificity of many of the now-routine preoperative tests. They then generated a case cost analysis for each of the tests based on standard charges for the test at the time and the screening of 1000 patients. As Table 13–4 shows, incredible amounts of money can be spent without significant results.

Based on this data and other information, the following recommendations are made for various tests.

(1) Hemoglobin/hematocrit: These tests for anemia are 100 per cent sensitive and specific, since the disorder is defined by the test itself. Because anemia is frequently asymptomatic and the added

**TABLE 13–3. Accuracy of Tests to Detect Asymptomatic Risk-Related Conditions**

| Test | Condition | Sensitivity (%) | Specificity (%) |
|------|-----------|-----------------|-----------------|
| ECG | Ischemic heart disease | 27 | 81 |
| Stress test | Ischemic heart disease | 64 | 91 |
| Partial thromboplastin time | Clotting disorder | 99 | 72 |
| Two-hour postprandial glucose | Diabetes | 76 | 56 |
| Tonometry (21 mm) | Glaucoma | 61 | 78 |
| SGOT | Hepatitis | 100 | 50 |
| Urine pregnancy test | Pregnancy | 98 | 99 |
| Purified protein derivative | Tuberculosis | 90 | 85 |
| Urine culture (voided) | Urinary tract infection | 95 | 84 |
| Hematocrit* | Anemia | 100 | 100 |
| Spirometry* | Chronic obstructive pulmonary disease | 100 | 100 |
| Platelet count* | Thrombocytopenia | 100 | 100 |
| Serum creatinine* | Renal disease | 100 | 100 |

*The abnormal test itself is used to define the presence or absence of the condition; therefore, sensitivity and specificity are considered to be 100%.
From Robbins JA, Mushlin AI: Preoperative evaluation of the healthy patient. Med Clin North Am 63:1145, 1979.

**TABLE 13–4. Consequences of Applying Tests to Determine Risk in a Asymptomatic Surgical Population of 1000 Patients**

| Test | Condition | Asymptomatic[a] Cases | Cases[b] Detected | Cases[b] Missed | False + Cases | Cost of[c] Testing | $ Cost/Case Found |
|---|---|---|---|---|---|---|---|
| Hematocrit | Anemia | 10 | 10 | 0 | 0 | $ 4,000 | 400 |
| ECG | Ischemic heart disease | 5 | 1 | 4 | 189 | 20,000 | 20,000 |
| Stress test | Ischemic heart disease | 5 | 3 | 2 | 90 | 150,000 | 50,000 |
| 24-hour monitor | Arrhythmias | 5 | 5 | | 0 | 179,000 | 35,800 |
| Spirometry | Chronic obstructive pulmonary disease | 19 | 19 | 0 | 0 | 22,500 | 4,500 |
| Two-hour postprandial glucose | Diabetes | 2.9 | 2 | 1 | 439 | 8,000 | 4,000 |
| Creatinine | Chronic renal disease | 0.3 | 0.3 | 0 | 0 | 9,000 | 30,000 |
| Partial thromboplastin time | Bleeding disorder | 0.01 | 0.01 | 0 | 280 | 11,000 | 1,100,000 |
| Platelet count | Thrombocytopenia | 0.05 | 0.05 | 0 | 0 | 7,000 | 140,000 |
| Urine protein | Nephrotic syndrome | 0.01 | 0.01 | 0 | ? | 3,000 | 300,000 |
| Chest x-ray | Interstitial lung disease | 0.1 | 0.1 | 0 | ? | 50,000 | 500,000 |
| Tonometry | Glaucoma | 0.2 | 0.1 | 0.1 | 220 | 12,250 | 122,500 |
| GC Culture | GC Female | 2.5 | 2. | 0 | ? | 18,000 | 7,200 |
| GC Smear | GC Male | 4.7 | 4.7 | 0 | ? | 7,000 | 1,489 |
| SGOT | Hepatitis | 0.25 | 0.25 | 0 | 500 | 9,000 | 36,000 |
| Urine pregnancy test | Pregnancy | 11 | 11 | 0 | 10 | 15,000 | 1,364 |
| RPR | Syphilis | 0.4 | 0.4 | 0.04 | ? | 10,000 | 25,000 |
| Purified protein derivative | Tuberculosis | 0.75 | 0.41 | 0.04 | 150 | 4,500 | 1,769 |
| Urine culture | ⎱ Bacteriuria and chronic renal disease | 14 | 13 | 1 | 158 | 23,000 | 1,769 |
| Urinalysis | ⎰ | 14 | 14 | 0 | ? | 5,000 | 357 |

[a] Based on prevalence of asymptomatic disease
[b] Based on sensitivity of each test
[c] Based on cost per test at University of Calfornia, Davis Medical Center per 1000 population tested

From Robbins JA, Mushlin AI: Preoperative evaluation of the healthy patient. Med Clin North Am 63:1145–1156, 1979.

blood loss secondary to surgery may severely compromise the patient, a screening hemoglobin or hematocrit should be performed on all surgical patients.

(2) Glucose: Galloway and Shuman[6] found, in 1963, that 24 per cent of the diabetics going to surgery were diagnosed on that admission. With the routine screening done on patients at the present time, the percentage is probably not as high. If the patient has had a blood glucose determination in the past one to two years, it need not be repeated. Otherwise, a serum fasting blood sugar should be done.

(3) Urinalysis: Because many medications are excreted through the kidneys and bladder catheterization occasionally is required, the status of renal function and the presence or absence of urinary pathogens should be determined preoperatively.

(4) Pregnancy testing should be performed on all females of childbearing age.

(5) ECG: Because of its low sensitivity, the ECG is not useful as a screening tool. In the 18-year followup[7] of the Framingham study, only 27 per cent of patients who suffered myocardial infarction had an abnormal ECG before the attack. However, a case can be made for use of the preoperative ECG as a comparison in those patients who are more at risk for ischemic heart disease based on age and family history if they should develop problems postoperatively. We therefore recommend it.

(6) Chest x-ray: The data are convincing that routine chest x-rays are not needed.

(7) Partial thromboplastin time: Unless the particular surgical procedure carries high risk for hemorrhage, routine screening of PTT need not be performed.

(8) SGOT: Measurement of SGOT is not necessary unless the patient belongs to a high-risk population (e.g., dialysis technician).

(9) Platelet count: Without signs or symptoms consistent with thrombocytopenia, routine measurement is not recommended.

A good argument can be made that the surgical period provides an excellent opportunity for periodic screening. In an extensive review of periodic healthy screening, Frame and Carlson[8] developed a flow sheet (Fig. 13–1) that provides an

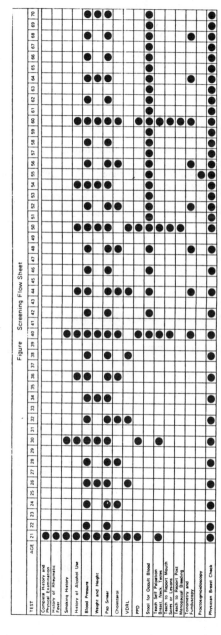

**Figure 13-1.** Screening flow chart. (From Frame PC, Carlsen SJ: A critical review of periodic health screening using specific screening criteria. J Fam Pract 2:289, 1975.)

excellent guide in this area. Consideration should be given to ordering the following tests based on the patient's need for healthy screening: cholesterol, VDRL (Venereal Disease Research Laboratories), purified protein derivative, stool for occult blood, Papanicolaou test, tonometry.

## REFERENCES

1. Committee on Records, American Society of Anesthesiologists Newsletter, No 27 (1971), p. 4.
2. Robbins J, Rose S: Partial thromboplastin time screening test. Ann Intern Med 90:796, 1979.
3. Bonebrake CR, Noller KL, Loehnen CP, et al: Routine chest roentgenography in pregnancy. JAMA 240:2747, 1978.
4. Robbins JA, Mushlin AI: Preoperative evaluation of the healthy patient. Med Clin North Am 63:1145, 1979.
5. Goldman L: Which tests are necessary for "healthy" patients? Consultants 24:331, 1984.
6. Galloway JA, Shuman CR: Diabetes and surgery. Am J Med 34:177, 1963.
7. Margolis JR, Kannel WB, Feinleib M: Clinical features of unrecognized myocardial infarction, patients and symptomatic, eighteen year follow-up, Framingham Study. Am J Cardiol 32:1, 1973.
8. Frame PS, Carlson SJ: A critical review of periodic health screening using specific screening criteria. J Fam Pract 2:29, 1975.

## II. NUTRITIONAL CARE

### A. PREOPERATIVE EVALUATION

1. Background and purpose

The prevalence of clinically significant protein-calorie malnutrition probably exceeds 15 per cent in many acute-care hospitals.[1] This is understandable when one takes into consideration the inadequate intake of nutrients with respect to metabolic demands of hospitalized patients. These patients become malnourished after admission as a result of catabolic stress and semistarvation regimens of 5% dextrose and water solutions. Elective and semielective surgical procedures can transform mild malnutrition into a clinically significant condition, in which immunodefense mechanisms are impaired, wound healing is delayed, and ultimate recovery is adversely affected.[2] The approach of the preoperative consultant should be to assess the nutritional parameters and advise a nutritional replacement regimen to reduce the morbidity and mortality of surgery.

2. Clinical assessment
   a. The history and physical examination for assessment of nutritional status were shown to be reproducible and valid by Baker and co-workers.[3]
      (1) History
         (a) Weight loss
         (b) Edema
         (c) Anorexia
         (d) Vomiting
         (e) Diarrhea
         (f) Decreased or unusual food intake
         (g) Chronic illness
      (2) Physical examination
         (a) Jaundice
         (b) Cheilosis
         (c) Glossitis
         (d) Loss of subcutaneous fat
         (e) Muscle wasting
         (f) Edema
   b. Figure 13–2 lists the major parameters for assessment of nutritional status.
   c. Anthropometric measurement includes the weight/height index, triceps skinfold thickness, arm muscle circumference, and creatinine/height index. These measurements are not sensitive enough alone to predict nutritional status in patients.
   d. Visceral proteins, such as albumin and transferrin, and delayed hypersensitivity can be easily assessed and have been correlated more accurately with morbidity and mortality. The probability of anergy, sepsis, and death with a given serum albumin is shown in Table 13–5.
   e. When deciding whether or not the patient should be treated with hyperalimentation, we use two methods of decision making.
      (1) Instant triple index of nutritional support[4, 5]

$$\left.\begin{array}{l}\text{albumin} <3.5 \text{ g\%} \\ \text{total lymphocyte} <1500 \text{ cu mm} \\ \text{absolute weight loss} >10 \text{ lbs}\end{array}\right\} \begin{array}{l}\text{should be} \\ \text{treated}\end{array}$$

      (2) Triple index of nutritional support (Table 13–6)
   f. Other methods of prognostication for nutritional status are listed in Tables 13–7 and 13–8. These methods are more involved and have not proved to be any more accurate than our triple assessment methods.

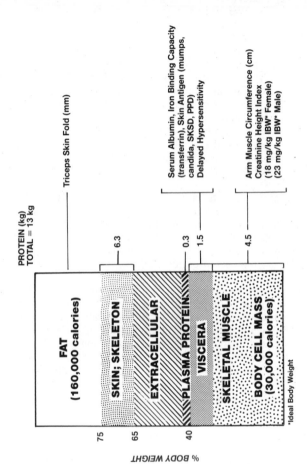

**Figure 13–2.** Major parameters for assessment of nutritional status. (From Blackburn GL, Bistrian BR, Maini BS, et al: Nutritional and metabolic assessment of the hospitalized patient. J Parenteral Enteral Nutrition *1*:11–22, 1977.)

**TABLE 13–5. Probability of Anergy, Sepsis, and Death at Given Serum Albumin Concentrations***

|        | <10% | <25% | 50% | >75% | >90% |
|--------|------|------|-----|------|------|
| Anergy | 5.2  | 4.2  | 3.2 | 2.2  | 1.2  |
| Sepsis | 4.3  | 3.7  | 3.1 | 2.5  | 1.9  |
| Death  | 4.9  | 4.0  | 3.2 | 2.3  | 1.5  |

*For example, a serum albumin concentration of 2.1 gm/dl is associated with a greater than 75 per cent estimated probability that anergy, sepsis, and death will occur during hospitalization.

From Blackburn GL, Harvey KB: Nutritional assessment as a routine in clinical medicine. Postgrad Med 71:46, 1982.

**TABLE 13–6. Guidelines to Assess Who Needs Nutritional Support**

| Baseline Nutritional Status | Severity of Actual or Anticipated Clinical Stress | Duration of Actual or Anticipated Starvation Before Initiation of Nutritional Support (Days) |
|---|---|---|
| Well nourished (ALB >3.5, TFN >220, DH reactive) | Moderate* | 7–10 |
| Well nourished | Severe† | 5–7 |
| Moderate malnutrition (ALB 3.0–3.5, TFN 180–220, DH reactive) | Moderate | 3–5 |
| Moderate malnutrition | Severe | 2–3 |
| Severe malnutrition (ALB <3, TFN <180, DH nonreactive) | Moderate or severe | <2 |

*For example, elective colon resection, biliary procedure, or thoracotomy.

†For example, combined thoracoabdominal procedure, hepatic resection, massive bowel resection or intraabdominal abscess.

Approximate guidelines for initiation of adjuvant nutritional support in surgical patients when there are no specific primary indications (e.g., inflammatory bowel disease, enteric fistula). The decision to initiate support is based on the patient's baseline nutritional status, severity of clinical stress, and period of actual or anticipated starvation. ALB = Serum albumin (gm/dl). TFN = Serum transferrin (mg/dl). DH = Skin test reactivity.

From Buzby GP Mullen JL: Nutrition and the surgical patient, in Goldmann DR, et al: Medical Care of the Surgical Patient, Philadelphia, JB Lippincott, 1982, pp 188–200.

**TABLE 13–7. Prognostic Nutritional Index**

PNI = 158% − 16.6 (Alb) − 0.78 (TSF) − 0.2 (TFN) − 5.8 (DH)

Alb = albumin in gm/dl
TSF = triceps skinfold in mm
TFN = transferrin in mg/dl
DH = delayed hypersensitivity

>5-mm induration = 2
1–5-mm induration = 1
anergy = 0

**Risk of Complication**
PNI ≥ 50% High
PNI = 40%–49% Intermediate
PNI ≤ 40% Low

From Mullen JL, Buzby G, Matthews DC, et al: Reduction of operative morbidity and mortality by combined preoperative and postoperative nutrition support. Ann Surg *192*:604–613, 1980.

## B. PERIOPERATIVE MANAGEMENT

1. Preoperative hyperalimentation

Our experience has been to start hyperalimentation five to ten days before the procedure when possible. If the surgery is urgent and there is less than five days, we recommend starting hyperalimentation after the surgery. The three studies listed in Table 13–9 indicate that preoperative hyperalimentation reduced the incidence of major infections and wound and anastomotic complications (morbidity) but did not reduce mortality.

2. Complications of total parenteral nutrition

**TABLE 13–8. Hospital Prognostic Index\***

HPI = 0.91 (Alb) − 1.00 (DH) 1.44 (sepsis) + 0.98 (diagnosis) − 1.09

Alb = albumin in gm/dl
DH = delayed hypersensitivity
≥5-mm induration = 1
anergy = 2

sepsis = 2; not septic = 1
Diagnosis: cancer = 1; not cancer = 2
  **Probability of Survival**
  HPI = 0 = 50%
  HPI = +1 = 74% } see graph
  HPI = −2 = 100%

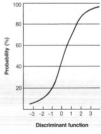

\*Adapted from Blackburn GL, Harvey KB: Nutritional assessment as a routine in clinical medicine. Nutr Assess *71*:62, 1982.

**TABLE 13–9. Effects of Preoperative Hyperalimentation**

| Study | Non-TPN | | TPN | | No. Days RX Preop |
|---|---|---|---|---|---|
| Mullen et al[6] | (95 pt) | 23% | (55 pt) | 4% | 7 days |
| Mueller et al[7] | ? | 32% | ? | 17% | 10 days |
| Daly et al[8] | (43 pt) | 23% | (72 pt) | 10% | 5 days |

    a. Mechanical[9]
      (1) Pneumothorax
      (2) Hemothorax
      (3) Catheter misplacement
      (4) Thrombosis
    b. Metabolic[10] (Table 13–10)
3. When hyperalimentation is being used, we recommend continuing the administration through the surgery. All patients should have pre-, intra-, and postoperative blood glucose and electrolytes measurements. These should be done daily until the patient is stable.
4. The total parenteral nutrition sheet illustrated in Figure 13–3 is used at our institution.
5. Management of complications
    a. Catheter[9]
      (1) Pneumothorax: Remove catheter; medical or surgical treatment.
      (2) Thrombosis: Remove catheter; add heparin to TPN.
      (3) Sepsis: Absolute removal with infection at entrance site, septicemia, or septic shock. Relative indications for removal are fever and inability to localize infection within 8 to 12 hours.
    b. Hypoglycemia:[10] Taper TPN infusion gradually.
    c. Hyperglycemia:[11] Add insulin to TPN or give peripherally.
    d. Hyperosmolar nonketotic hyperglycemia:[12, 13] Slow or stop TPN, insulin; manage fluid and electrolytes.
    e. Metabolic acidosis (hyperchloremic):[14] Decrease NaCl in solution and substitute Na acetate.
    f. Hypokalemia:[11] Administer supplemental potassium.
    g. Hypophosphatemia:[11] Administer 7 to 10 mmoles per 1000 kcal.
    h. Hypomagnesemia:[11] Give 0.35 to 0.45 mEq/kg/day as magnesium sulfate.

**TABLE 13–10. Metabolic Complications of Total Parenteral Nutrition**

| Problems | Possible Etiologies |
| --- | --- |
| GLUCOSE METABOLISM | |
| Hyperglycemia, glycosuria, osmotic diuresis, hyperosmolar nonketotic dehydration and coma | Excessive total dose or rate of infusion of glucose, inadequate endogenous insulin |
| Ketoacidosis in diabetes mellitus | Inadequate endogenous insulin response; inadequate exogenous insulin therapy |
| Postinfusion hypoglycemia | Persistence of endogenous insulin production secondary to prolonged stimulation of islet cells by high-carbohydrate infusion |
| AMINO ACID METABOLISM | |
| Hyperchloremic metabolic acidosis | Excessive chloride and monohydrochloride content of crystalline amino acid solutions |
| Serum amino acid imbalances | Unphysiologic amino acid profile of the nutrient solution |
| Hyperammonemia | Excessive ammonia in protein hydrolysate solutions; arginine, ornithine, aspartic acid, or glutamic acid deficiency in amino acid solutions; primary hepatic disorder |
| Prerenal azotemia | Excessive protein hydrolysate or amino acid infusion |
| CALCIUM AND PHOSPHORUS METABOLISM | |
| Hypophosphatemia | Inadequate phosphorus administration; redistribution of serum phosphorus into cells or bone |

| | |
|---|---|
| —Decreased erythrocyte 2,3-diphosphoglycerate | |
| —Increased affinity of hemoglobin for oxygen | |
| —Aberrations of erythrocyte intermediary metabolites | |
| Hypocalcemia | Inadequate calcium administration; reciprocal response to phosphorus repletion without simultaneous calcium infusion |
| Hypercalcemia | Excessive calcium administration with or without high dose of albumin |
| Vitamin D deficiency; hypervitaminosis D | Inadequate or excessive vitamin D administration |
| ESSENTIAL FATTY ACID METABOLISM | |
| Serum deficiencies of phospholipid linoleic or arachidonic acids; serum elevations of 5,8,11-eicosatrienoic acid | Inadequate essential fatty acid administration; inadequate vitamin E administration |
| MISCELLANEOUS | |
| Hypokalemia to increased requirements for protein | Inadequate potassium intake relative in anabolism |
| Hyperkalemia | Excessive potassium administration, especially in metabolic acidosis |
| Hypomagnesemia | Inadequate magnesium administration relative to increased requirements for protein anabolism |
| Anemia | Iron deficiency; folic acid deficiency; vitamin $B_{12}$ deficiency; copper deficiency |
| Bleeding | Vitamin K deficiency |
| Hypervitaminosis A | Excessive vitamin A administration |
| Elevations in SGOT, SGPT, and serum alkaline phosphatase | Enzyme induction secondary to accelerated glucose metabolism, possible hepatotoxicity secondary to amino acid imbalance; excessive glycogen or fat deposition in the liver |

From Dudrick SJ, MacFedyen BV, Van Buren CT, et al: Parenteral hyperalimentation, metabolic problems and solutions. Ann Surg 179:259, 1972.

**DAILY ADULT PARENTERAL NUTRITION**
**PHYSICIAN'S TREATMENT SHEET**
**THOMAS JEFFERSON UNIVERSITY HOSPITAL**

Name _____

Room _____

MR# _____

X No. _____

Doctor _____

"Authorization is hereby given to dispense a chemically identical drug (as recommended by the Pharmacy & Therapeutics Committee) unless the 'Request for Non-Formulary Drug' form is completed and submitted for the information of the Pharmacy & Therapeutics Committee."

ALLERGIES:

COMPLETE ABOVE OR IMPRINT WITH ADDRESSOPLATE

This form is for Parenteral Nutrition (**PN**) Orders only. Requests for repeat of previous day's orders are not acceptable. Orders must be written daily and received by the Pharmacy by **10 A.M.**

| | | Nursing Noted |
|---|---|---|
| **ORDER** Check appropriate box in each section. | | |
| ☒ | **ROUTINE PROCEDURES** (All **PN** patients): Strict Intake/Output; Daily weights; Catheter for **PN** use only; Monitor pump function and flow rate. | |
| | Urine fractionals every 6 hours<br>☐ +3 obtain stat serum glucose  ☐ +3 _____ units of regular insulin sc  ☐ +4 _____ units of regular insulin sc; | |
| ☐ | **BASELINE VALUES** (to be obtained on first day of **PN**) — CBC with Diff.; PT; PTT; BUN; glucose; electrolytes; SMA$_{12}$; Mg; TIBC and Serum Iron. Weight. | |
| | **LABORATORY MONITORING** | |
| ☐ | **INITIAL MONITORING** (recommended until stable) — Daily; vital signs every 4 hours; BUN; glucose; electrolytes.<br>Mon. & Thurs.: SMA$_{12}$, Serum Mg, CBC with diff. | |
| ☐ | **STABLE MONITORING** Mon. & Thurs.: BUN; glucose; electrolytes; SMA$_{12}$; Mon.: Serum Mg; TIBC | |
| | **OPTIONAL TESTS**<br>☐ 24 hr. Urine (creatinine and urea nitrogen)  ☐ Serum Folate  ☐ Serum B$_{12}$  ☐ Serum Fe | |
| ☐ | Check Box for **RATE CHANGE** on PN to become effective immediately. | |

PRINT IN THIS SPACE

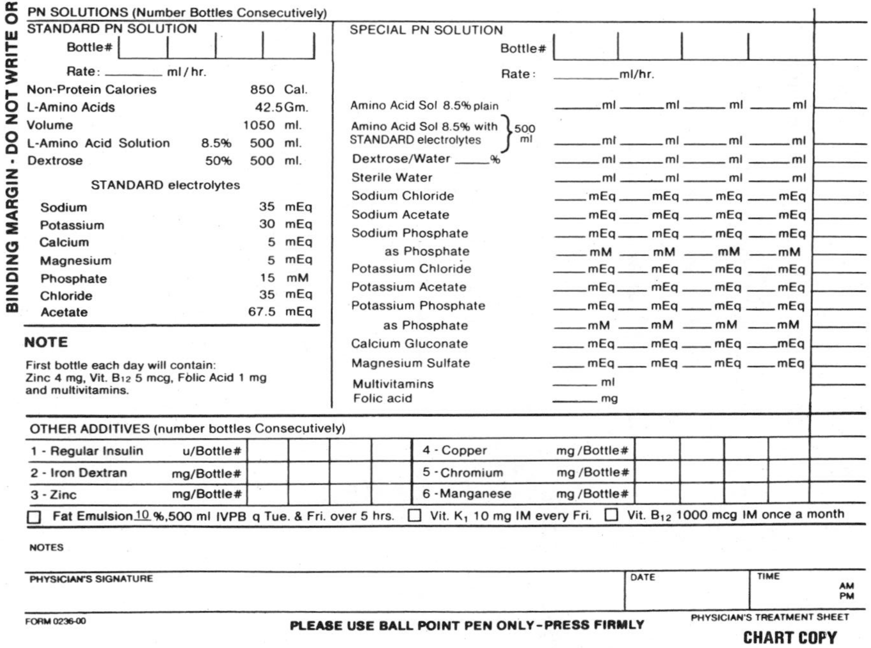

BINDING MARGIN - DO NOT WRITE OR

PN SOLUTIONS (Number Bottles Consecutively)

**STANDARD PN SOLUTION**

Bottle# | | | | |

Rate: ______ ml / hr.

| | | | |
|---|---|---|---|
| Non-Protein Calories | | 850 | Cal. |
| L-Amino Acids | | 42.5 | Gm. |
| Volume | | 1050 | ml. |
| L-Amino Acid Solution | 8.5% | 500 | ml. |
| Dextrose | 50% | 500 | ml. |

STANDARD electrolytes

| | | |
|---|---|---|
| Sodium | 35 | mEq |
| Potassium | 30 | mEq |
| Calcium | 5 | mEq |
| Magnesium | 5 | mEq |
| Phosphate | 15 | mM |
| Chloride | 35 | mEq |
| Acetate | 67.5 | mEq |

**NOTE**

First bottle each day will contain:
Zinc 4 mg, Vit. $B_{12}$ 5 mcg, Folic Acid 1 mg
and multivitamins.

**SPECIAL PN SOLUTION**

Bottle# | | | | |

Rate: ______ ml/hr.

| | | | | |
|---|---|---|---|---|
| Amino Acid Sol 8.5% plain | ____ ml | ____ ml | ____ ml | ____ ml |
| Amino Acid Sol 8.5% with STANDARD electrolytes } 500 ml | ____ ml | ____ ml | ____ ml | ____ ml |
| Dextrose/Water ____ % | ____ ml | ____ ml | ____ ml | ____ ml |
| Sterile Water | ____ ml | ____ ml | ____ ml | ____ ml |
| Sodium Chloride | ____ mEq | ____ mEq | ____ mEq | ____ mEq |
| Sodium Acetate | ____ mEq | ____ mEq | ____ mEq | ____ mEq |
| Sodium Phosphate | ____ mEq | ____ mEq | ____ mEq | ____ mEq |
| as Phosphate | ____ mM | ____ mM | ____ mM | ____ mM |
| Potassium Chloride | ____ mEq | ____ mEq | ____ mEq | ____ mEq |
| Potassium Acetate | ____ mEq | ____ mEq | ____ mEq | ____ mEq |
| Potassium Phosphate | ____ mEq | ____ mEq | ____ mEq | ____ mEq |
| as Phosphate | ____ mM | ____ mM | ____ mM | ____ mM |
| Calcium Gluconate | ____ mEq | ____ mEq | ____ mEq | ____ mEq |
| Magnesium Sulfate | ____ mEq | ____ mEq | ____ mEq | ____ mEq |
| Multivitamins | ____ ml | | | |
| Folic acid | ____ mg | | | |

OTHER ADDITIVES (number bottles Consecutively)

| | | | | | | | | | | | |
|---|---|---|---|---|---|---|---|---|---|---|---|
| 1 - Regular Insulin | u/Bottle# | | | | | 4 - Copper | mg /Bottle# | | | | |
| 2 - Iron Dextran | mg/Bottle# | | | | | 5 - Chromium | mg /Bottle# | | | | |
| 3 - Zinc | mg/Bottle# | | | | | 6 - Manganese | mg /Bottle# | | | | |

☐ Fat Emulsion 10 %,500 ml IVPB q Tue. & Fri. over 5 hrs. ☐ Vit. $K_1$ 10 mg IM every Fri. ☐ Vit. $B_{12}$ 1000 mcg IM once a month

NOTES

PHYSICIAN'S SIGNATURE | DATE | TIME AM PM

FORM 0236-00

**PLEASE USE BALL POINT PEN ONLY - PRESS FIRMLY**

PHYSICIAN'S TREATMENT SHEET

**CHART COPY**

**Figure 13–3.** Parenteral nutrition treatment sheet.

   i. Hypocalcemia:[11] Give 0.2 to 0.3 mEq/kg/day as calcium glucose.

   j. Essential fatty acid deficiency:[15, 16] 500 ml of 10% essential fatty acids twice weekly.

   k. Trace mineral deficiency[17, 18, 19]
     (1) Zinc: 3 mg/day
     (2) Copper: 1.6 mg/day
     (3) Manganese: 2 to 3 mg/day or 0.006 mEq/kg/day
     (4) Iodide: 1 µg/kg/day

   l. Vitamins:[11] Vitamin $B_{12}$ 100 µg once per month IM; folic acid 1 mg/day; multivitamins once per day

  m. Hypoprothrombinemia:[11] Vitamin K 10 mg once per week

   n. Liver function:[20, 21, 22, 23] Lower glucose content and reassess.

   o. Prerenal azotemia:[10, 14] Evaluate hydration.

## REFERENCES

1. Blackburn GL, Harvey KB: Nutritional assessment as a routine in clinical medicine. Postgrad Med *71*:46, 1982.
2. Bistrian BR, Blackburn GL, Scrimshaw NS, et al: Cellular immunity in semistarved states in hospitalized adults. Am J Clin Nutr *218*:1148, 1975.
3. Baker JP, Detsky AS, Wesson DE, et al: Nutritional assessment: A comparison of clinical judgement and objective measurements. N Engl J Med *306*:969, 1982.
4. Seltzer MH, Fletcher HS, Slocum BA, et al: Instant nutritional assessment in the intensive care unit. J Parenteral Enteral Nutrition *5*:70, 1981.
5. Seltzer MH, Slocum BA, Cataldi-Betcher EL: Instant nutritional assement: Absolute weight loss and surgical mortality. J Parenteral Enteral Nutrition *6*:218, 1982.
6. Mullen JL, Buzby GP, Matthews DC, et al: Reduction of operative morbidity and mortality by combined preoperative and postoperative nutritional support. Ann Surg *192*:604, 1980.
7. Mueller JM, Dienst C, Brenner U, et al: Perioperative TPN in patients with upper gastrointestinal malignancies. Lancet *1*:68, 1981.
8. Daly JM, Massar E, Giacco G: Parenteral nutrition in esophageal cancer patients. Ann Surg *196*:203, 1982.
9. Sheldon GF, Baker C: Complications of nutritional support. Crit Care Med *8*:35, 1980.
10. Dudrick SJ, MacFedyen BV, VanBuren CT, et al: Parenteral hyperalimentation, metabolic problems and solutions. Ann Surg *179*:259, 1972.
11. Fischer JE: Total parenteral nutrition. Boston, Little, Brown, 1976.
12. Sanderson I, Deitel M: Insulin response in patients receiving

concentrated infusions of glucose and casein hydrolysate for complete parenteral nutrition. Ann Surg *179*:387, 1974.

13. Doromal NM, Canter JW: Hyperosmolar hyperglycemic nonketotic coma complicating intravenous hyperalimentation. Surg Gynecol Obstet *136*:729, 1973.

14. Myers RN, Smink RD, Goldstein F: Parenteral hyperalimentation, five years' clinical experience. Am J Gastroenterol *62*:313, 1974.

15. Faulkner WJ, Flint LM: Essential fatty acid deficiency associated with total parenteral nutrition. Surg Gynecol Obstet *144*:665, 1977.

16. McCarthy DM, May RJ, Maher M, et al: Trace metal and essential fatty acid deficiency during total parenteral nutrition. Am J Dig Dis *23*:1009, 1978.

17. Lowry SF, Goodgame JT, Smith JC, et al: Abnormalities of zinc and copper during total parenteral nutrition. Ann Surg *189*:120, 1979.

18. Kay RG, Tasman-Jones C, Pybus J, et al.: A syndrome of acute zinc deficiency during total parenteral alimentation in man. Ann Surg *183*:331, 1976.

19. Jeegeebhoy KN, Chu RC, Marliss EB, et al: Chromium deficiency, glucose intolerance and neuropathy reversed by chromium supplementation in a patient receiving long-term parenteral nutrition. Am J Clin Nutr *30*:531, 1977.

20. Rodgers BM, Hollenbeck JI, Donnelly WH, et al: Intrahepatic cholestasis with parenteral alimentation. Am J Surg *131*:149, 1976.

21. Grant JP, Kleinman LM, Maher MM, et al: Serum hepatic enzyme and bilirubin elevations during parenteral nutrition. Surg Gynecol Obstet *145*:573, 1977.

22. Touloukina RJ, Downing SE: Cholestasis associated with long-term parenteral alimentation. Arch Surg *106*:58, 1973.

23. Sheldon GF, Peterson SR, Sanders R: Hepatic dysfunction during hyperalimentation. Arch Surg *113*:504, 1978.

## III. THE ORTHOPEDIC/RHEUMATOLOGIC PATIENT

# FRACTURES

Frequently, there are multiple systemic injuries in addition to the known fractures. These multiple injuries must be evaluated comprehensively by the medical/surgical team.

Lacerations and soft-tissue injuries should receive appropriate treatment. Hematomas should be evaluated, and if there is a suggestion of a complicating infection, they must be aspirated. Open wounds from trauma requiring surgery often become infected, as do open fractures and open joint wounds. Prophylactic antibiotics should be considered. Short courses of prophylactic antibiotics with soft-tissue injury and fractures or open fractures may reduce postoperative infection rate by 50 per cent.[1]

In total joint replacement, short courses of antistaphylococcal antibiotics in the form of nafcillin or other antistaphylococcal drugs, such as cephalothin, given up to 12 hours preoperatively and up to 48 hours postoperatively have been shown in some cases to reduce postoperative infection from the staphylococcus by 50 per cent. The use of prophylactic antibiotics is adjunctive to good operative technique and careful skin cleansing.

In hip fracture, prophylactic antibiotics have been shown, in some series, to reduce postoperative infection, although the result is not as dramatic as in total joint replacement.

In "clean" orthopedic surgery—that is, procedures not involving trauma or the insertion of a prosthesis—it is difficult to show a beneficial effect of prophylactic antibiotics.

## THE HIP

Controversy remains as to whether patients with total hip replacement or repair of hip fractures should receive anticoagulants. Such patients seem to have little, if any, benefit from standard low-dose heparin prophylaxis, based on multiple studies.[2, 3] However, a recent study by Leyvraz and others[4] provides evidence that one can significantly reduce the incidence of thrombophlebitis after hip replacement surgery by adjusting the dosage of prophylactic subcutaneous heparin to yield partial thromboplastin time in the high-normal range, thereby restoring normal hemostatic equilibrium.

Aspirin has been shown in at least one study to decrease postoperative deep venous thrombosis in men undergoing orthopedic procedures but not in women.[5]

Alternative methods to prevent deep venous thrombosis, such as the use of supportive stockings, early ambulation, and isometric exercise, should be seriously considered.

## PREOPERATIVE EVALUATION OF THE PATIENT WITH JOINT DISEASE

In the patient with rheumatoid arthritis who has symptoms referable to the neck, it is considered standard practice to obtain neck x-rays with flexion and extension views to exclude atlanto-axial subluxation. Patients with atlanto-axial subluxation are prone to spinal cord injury during the operative procedure when the head is fully extended for insertion of an endotracheal tube.

Patients with rheumatoid arthritis may also have temporomandibular joint dysfunction and difficulty opening the mouth. Patients with a combination of neck and jaw disease are even more likely to have difficulty with establishing an airway in the beginning of the anesthesia.

# PREOPERATIVE EVALUATION OF THE PATIENT WITH SYSTEMIC LUPUS ERYTHEMATOSUS

Patients taking corticosteroids should be continued in the same dosage. Patients with active disease may have an exacerbation of their disease precipitated by the surgery and anesthesia, and this may require an increased dosage of corticosteroids postoperatively. Preoperatively, the patient should have the usual medical assessment, as well as careful evaluation of those organ systems known to have been involved with the disease in the past. If there is asymptomatic progression, studies should be obtained to evaluate renal function. Chest x-ray, ECG, and echocardiography may be needed to evaluate a suspected pleural effusion or pericardial effusion.

Patients with dermatomyositis, polymyositis, temporal arteritis, or polymyalgia rheumatica who have been steroid-dependent should have their steroids continued and, if the disease is active, should have the corticosteroids raised to pharmacologic levels during and shortly after the surgical procedure. Their corticosteroids could be raised to the equivalent of 60 mg of prednisone a day for one to two weeks and then tapered rapidly to the preoperative levels.

Patients with scleroderma (progressive systemic sclerosis) should have careful clinical evaluation of the heart, lungs, and kidneys. Because corticosteroid therapy is not usually beneficial, it should not be initiated preoperatively but should be continued if the patient is currently taking this medication.

# DEGENERATIVE JOINT DISEASE

Those patients having elective surgery of the chest or abdomen who have symptoms referable to peripheral joints involved with osteoarthritis, such as fingers, hips, and knees, should have physical protection and symptomatic therapy of the joints in the immediate perioperative period. Those patients having symptomatic involvement of the spine should have protection of that area with careful movement on and off the operating table and symptomatic treatment in the form of non-steroidal analgesic agents. It is seldom necessary to delay surgery for symptomatic treatment of degenerative joint disease since treatment procedures for these entities are relatively unsatisfactory.

## REFERENCES

1. Lindgren L, et al: Orthopedic infection during a 5-year period, 1963-1967. Acta Orthop Scand *43*:325, 1972.
2. Hampson WGJ, Harris FC, Lucas HK, et al: Failure of low-dose heparin to prevent deep-vein thrombosis after hip-replacement arthroplasty. Lancet *2*:795–797, 1974.
3. Sikorski JM, Hampson WG, Staddon GE: The natural history of aetiology of deep-vein thrombosis after total hip-replacement. J Bone Joint Surg *63*:171–177, 1981.
4. Leyvraz PF, Richard J, Bachman F, et al: Adjusted versus fixed-dose subcutaneous heparin in the prevention of deep-vein thrombosis after total hip-replacement. N Engl J Med *309*:954–958, 1983.
5. Harris WH, Salzman EW, Athanosoulis CA, et al: Aspirin prophylaxis of venous thromboembolism after total hip-replacement. N Engl J Med *297*:1246–1249, 1977.

## IV. THE ORAL SURGERY PATIENT

# DENTAL SURGERY

The physician should always be aware that during dental surgery the operative procedure is taking place through the airway so that any previous compromise of the airway may be magnified owing to local manipulation or bleeding.

Patients presenting for emergency surgery for nondental procedures should have the mouth, head, and neck evaluated before surgery. Those patients with symptomatic dental problems may need oral surgical consultation before elective surgery in order to prevent complications. Signs and symptoms suggesting serious oral disease are painful chewing, previous dental problems, teeth sensitive to hot or cold, difficulty opening the mouth, mouth or throat pain, and an enlarged tongue.[1]

Physical examination of the oral cavity may show evidence of dental caries, loose teeth, temporomandibular joint dysfunction, periodontal abscess, or acute and subacute infections of the mouth, gums, and teeth. These problems can contribute to anesthesic morbidity by manipulation and trauma to these diseased structures with the insertion of the laryngoscope.

Dental plates should be noted and removed before the operative procedure. All patients with juvenile rheumatoid arthritis should be suspected of having temporomandibular joint dysfunction, as should most patients with adult rheumatoid arthritis. Some patients who are to undergo prosthetic heart valve surgery should have specific treatment of severely decayed teeth with, perhaps, extractions before a prosthetic heart valve is inserted to minimize the possibility of postoperative endocarditis. All should receive antibiotic prophylaxis.

If there is infection around à partially erupted third molar in young adults, elective systemic surgery should be delayed until infection can be cleared with penicillin or other antibiotics and, perhaps, definitive treatment of the infected molar area.

Temporomandibular joint problems in patients with rheumatoid arthritis and juvenile rheumatoid arthritis have previously been noted. Many patients with temporomandibular joint pain have pain that cannot be explained on the basis of trauma or inflammatory joint disease. The pain is frequently idiopathic, but this must be noted before elective systemic surgery.

## JAW HYPOMOBILITY

Patients with difficulty opening their mouths for whatever reason should have this abnormality noted before elective surgery. Such patients may need dental consultation before elective surgery. In the event of emergency surgery, the anesthesiologist must be forewarned of this abnormality.

## SALIVARY GLAND DISEASE

Salivary gland neoplasms usually are evidenced by tumor in the gland itself.

Acute postoperative parotitis may occur related to dehydration in elderly or debilitated postoperative patients. This is a serious and sometimes life-threatening illness that requires prompt treatment with IV antibiotics having antistaphylococcal spectrum.

## REFERENCE

1. Kaban, LB: Dental and oral surgical problems in the preoperative Patient, in Vandam LD (ed): To Make the Patient Ready for Anesthesia. Menlo Park, California, Addison-Wesley, 1980, pp 202–217.

## V. THE OPHTHALMOLOGIC PATIENT

Consulting physicians are often asked to evaluate and care for patients undergoing ocular surgery. Few data are available on the preoperative evaluation of these patients. In many cases it is reasonable to apply the principles used for general surgery; in some areas, however, there are fundamental differences that require specific knowledge of ocular disease and therapy.

### A. RISK ASSESSMENT—MEDICAL RISKS

1. Indications for general anesthesia

    Although the majority of ophthalmic surgical procedures can be done under local blocks, surgeons may request general anesthesia. This is true for various reasons. They may be concerned about patients moving during a delicate procedure. Being perfectly still for several hours may be difficult for even the most cooperative patient. Some patients with hearing or mental impairment or language difficulties may not be able to follow instructions and could move at a critical time. Other reasons for using general anesthesia include a bleeding diathesis, increasing the risk of a retro-orbital hemorrhage; an allergy to local anesthetic or poor results with the local block; or the patient's own apprehension about the surgical procedure.

2. Anesthesia in relation to ophthalmic risk

    Using general anesthesia when a local block could be used presents a problem for the medical consultant. Typically, one regards the risk of local anesthesia to be less than that of general anesthesia. Despite this, the consultant is often asked to "clear" the patient for general anesthesia. In such cases the physician must consider the ocular risks as well as the medical risks. There is no formula for this assessment, but one must consider the type and difficulty of the surgery, the threat to the vision, and even the skill of the surgeon and anesthesiologist. It may be inappropriate to give clearance for general anesthesia for a patient with a compromised cardiopulmonary system when an extremely slow surgeon plans a long procedure, such as a posterior vitrectomy. On the other hand, greater risks must be accepted when there is an imminent threat to sight. In retinal detachments in which there is danger of losing macular vision, all but the most unusual risks may be accepted. This is especially true in cases in which vision is impaired in the opposite eye. When there is little hope of recovering useful vision, one should be more conservative. Naturally, these assessments must be made in consultation with the ophthalmologist.

3. Mortality with ocular surgery

   The mortality for ocular surgery has been reported to range from 0.06 per cent to 0.18 per cent.[1,2] Although this may vary with such factors as type of surgery and age, the most accurate estimates of overall mortality in which some aspect of hospitalization contributed to death are 0.10 per cent to 0.13 per cent.[3]

   a. General vs. local anesthesia: In review of 47,000 patients at the Wilmer Institute, Quigley[3] found older patients to fare less well under general anesthesia, whereas for younger patients there was no mortality difference between general and local. It is important to note that in this study, there is no significant difference in the mortality per case for the two types of anesthesia. However, the average age of the patients receiving local anesthesia was greater than that of patients receiving general anesthesia. It is also likely that for high-risk patients, ocular surgery is done more often under local. If this is true, equal mortality rates would suggest that local anesthesia is actually safer. Other authors have reported death rates associated with general and local anesthesia in ophthalmic surgery to be equal,[1] over twice as high for general,[4] and twice as high for local.[5] The question of relative risk is difficult to resolve because of different methods of data collection (questionnaires, chart reviews, and perspective studies), the need for large numbers, and the incomplete data about the medical condition of patients in each group. For example, Wolfe and co-workers[6] have reported a mortality of only 0.05 per cent with general anesthesia. Although this is much better than most reviews, the study included only 2217 patients. One additional death in this group would have made the average 0.10 per cent, exactly equal to the general average.

   b. Medical disease in relation to mortality risk: Petruscak

**TABLE 13–11. Incidence of Mortality in Ophthalmic Surgery**

| Type of Surgery | % Mortality | Relative Risk |
| --- | --- | --- |
| All patients | 0.1 | 1.0 |
| Muscle surgery | 0.10 | 0.1 |
| Retinal detachment | 0.24 | 2.4 |

From Quigley HA: Mortality associated with ophthalmic surgery: A twenty-year experience at Wilmer Institute. Am J Ophthalmol 77:517, 1974.

and associates[4] reported mortality to be twice as high for local anesthesia as for general in 17,155 patients at the Eye and Ear Hospital in Pittsburgh. More important, these authors found 1 death in the ASA Class II (moderate systemic disturbance), 18 deaths in ASA Class III (severe systemic disturbance), and no deaths in ASA Class I (healthy). Only three of these deaths occurred intraoperatively.

c. Ocular disease in relation to mortality risk: Although underlying medical factors are probably the most important consideration, other factors are also associated with higher mortality. In the study by Quigley,[3] patients undergoing retinal detachment surgery have over twice the mortality of cataract patients, despite being ten years younger on the average. Patients undergoing muscle surgery, who were much younger than retinal detachment patients, had only one twentieth the mortality of retinal detachment, despite an equal frequency of general anesthesias (Table 13–11).[3]

Although there is no explanation for this difference, the retinal detachment patients had more underlying medical problems and had a longer postoperative period of bed rest than the other two groups.

d. Fatality in ophthalmologic patients

(1) Pulmonary embolism as most common cause: Kaplan and Reba[5] reviewed 21,400 ophthalmic inpatient procedures and found 30 deaths. Of the 19 patients who underwent autopsy, 9 (43 per cent) died of pulmonary emboli. In only two cases was the diagnosis made clinically. Of the 11 cases who did not undergo autopsy, none had a clinical diagnosis of pulmonary embolism. Myocardial infarction was the most common clinical diagnosis in cases in which a pulmonary embolus was proven by autopsy to be the cause of death. Seven of the

19 patients had negative medical histories. Of these, five of seven had retinal detachments, four of seven died of pulmonary emboli, and two of seven had complications of general anesthesia.

(2) Risk of prior myocardial infarction: a study by Backer and others[7] from the Mayo Clinic attempts to evaluate the influence of myocardial infarction on the risk of ophthalmic surgery. These authors reviewed 280 ophthalmic operations on patients who had had previous myocardial infarctions and found no episodes of reinfarctions. This is in contrast to the 6.1 per cent reinfarction rate seen in general surgery and the 3.6 per cent reinfarction rate found even when high-risk procedures were deleted from general anesthesia.[8] Unfortunately, all but 27 of these procedures were done under local block, precluding a reliable assessment of reinfarction risk for ocular surgery under general anesthesia. However, the risk of reinfarction for ocular surgery under local anesthesia is low.

4. Conclusions

Several conclusions can be drawn from the above information:

a. The underlying systemic problems are the most important determinant of medical risk.

b. For general anesthesia, old age, underlying medical problems, and retinal detachment surgery probably all enhance medical risks.

c. For younger patients, there is little additional risk with general anesthesia.

d. In patients with a history of myocardial infarction and who are medically stable, there is a minimal reinfarction rate when local anesthesia is used.

e. The overall risk of ocular surgery is so low that even patients with serious systemic conditions should be candidates for elective surgery if there is sufficient opportunity to restore sight.

## B. RISK ASSESSMENT—OCULAR RISK

A physician who is evaluating a patient for eye surgery must also be concerned with ocular risk. Certain conditions, although not medically serious, may pose a threat to vision even though they represent little threat to the patient.

1. Cough

Probably the most important ocular risk is cough. The patient with a persistent cough, owing to such factors as smoking, allergies, or a recent bronchitis, may be at little systemic risk for something as simple as ocular surgery. However, if the cough cannot be controlled in surgery, the pressure transmitted to an eye that has been surgically opened could expel its contents and destroy the eye. Therefore, it is important to inform the anesthesiologist and the surgeon of even a mild, persistent cough and to make every effort to correct its cause. A correctible cause for persistent cough may be reason to delay elective surgery.

2. Blood pressure

    Diastolic blood pressures below 110 have not been found to increase mortality in general surgery.[9] However, high blood pressures, especially in diabetics undergoing vitrectomy, may increase the risk of bleeding into the eye. One should be more aggressive with antihypertensive therapy when ophthalmic vascular surgery is planned.

3. Bleeding problems

    We have seen several cases of serious retrobulbar hemorrhage in patients taking aspirin who have a prolonged bleeding time, as well as in one patient with advanced liver disease and abnormalities of prothrombin time. Although we have also seen many patients with both liver disease and prolonged bleeding times undergo cataract surgery without incident, it seems most prudent to correct bleeding parameters before surgery whenever possible. One exception to this might be noted: Hall and Steen[10] have reported uncomplicated cataract surgery in 16 eyes of 13 patients who were fully anticoagulated with warfarin so that the prothrombin times were twice that of control values. We have noted one episode of bleeding from retrobulbar block that required rescheduling of surgery in an anticoagulated patient but presented no serious threat to the eye. We have seen no bleeding complications from the cataract surgery itself in the anticoagulated patients. Although we still believe in stopping anticoagulation when possible, cataract surgery can be performed safely in anticoagulated patients when the risk of reversal is high. Although general anesthesia is recommended in most cases, retrobulbar block can be done if sufficient time is permitted after the block to be sure that no retro-orbital bleeding has occurred.

4. Infection

    One final ocular risk factor is infection elsewhere in the body. Postoperative eyes are vulnerable to infection for many reasons:

   a. Sutures and foreign bodies from the surgery
   b. A poor blood supply and poor defense mechanisms
   c. Only a mild amount of inflammation and scarring may
      cause serious impairment of vision
   d. A tendency for the patient to unconsciously rub the
      irritated eye
         Any superficial infection can be unconsciously in-
      oculated into the eye, causing infection and scarring.
      In these patients, it is as important to check for areas
      of superficial infection as it is to ask about symptoms
      of systemic infections.

## C. MEDICAL PROBLEMS IN EYE PATIENTS

   1. Fluid and electrolyte imbalance
         Certain problems occur more frequently in eye patients
      because of the population seen and their medical prob-
      lems and medications. The most common of these med-
      ical complications are dehydration and electrolyte imbal-
      ance, which occur primarily in older patients receiving
      thiazide or loop diuretics. In addition to the diuretics,
      four factors contribute to this condition. The most im-
      portant of these is the use of mannitol preoperatively to
      reduce intraocular tension, as well as the use of aceta-
      zolamide postoperatively for the same reason. Both of
      these diuretics act to enhance the action of the loop and
      distal agents and markedly increase potassium, sodium,
      and water excretion. In addition to this, the naturetic
      affect of bed rest and the reduction in intake because of
      surgical routine, as well as the nausea produced by high
      ocular pressures, pain, and the acetazolamide itself, can
      combine to produce marked dehydration. The physician
      will be called to see a patient two or three days postop-
      eratively who is weak, listless, and light-headed when
      standing. The blood pressure is normal or low and nearly
      always drops lower with sitting or standing. When this
      condition is recognized, a diuretic or acetazolamide must
      be stopped and fluid and electrolytes replaced. This may
      be done by formulation, such as Pedialyte or Gatorade,
      or by IV replacement. We have trained the nurses who
      take care of eye patients to notify the ophthalmologist
      or medical consultant if acetazolamide is started in a
      patient already on a diuretic. It is usually a prudent
      preventive measure to stop the diuretic when this occurs.
      Finally, patients who are admitted on a combination of
      acetazolamide and another diuretic should always be
      checked for hypokalemia.

2. Problems seen in diabetics
   a. Two less common problems involve diabetics. In cyclocryotherapy, a probe, cooled with liquid nitrogen, is used to freeze the area around the limbus to reduce the production of vitreous humor. Although this is a bedside procedure and does not require that the patient have an empty stomach, there is a high incidence of nausea and vomiting afterward. Patients who have had their full dose of insulin may develop hypoglycemia owing to the inability to eat.
   b. The second problem involves diabetics who are being maintained on acetazolamide. This agent's bicarbonate-wasting action permits less buffer to be available if these patients should become ketotic. This may be a problem in patients with a preexisting renal tubular acidosis, which is sometimes seen in diabetics. It may be necessary to give oral or even parenteral bicarbonate to such patients.
3. The "full bladder syndrome"
   The "full bladder syndrome" is common in ophthalmic patients. The most common setting is an elderly male who develops marked hypertension postoperatively. The hypertension might be quite refractory to therapy. On examination, one finds a markedly distended bladder, probably related to the preoperative use of mannitol. Catheterization is therapeutic. However, if any hypertensive medication was given before noticing the bladder distention, hypotension may occur after catheterization. When postoperative hypertension is new or out of proportion to preoperative levels, one should check for bladder distention before administering antihypertensive drugs.
4. Systemic effects of eye drops
   The systemic effects of eye drops must not be overlooked. This subject has been reviewed by us and will be only briefly discussed here.[11, 12] Systemic absorption of drops occurs through the conjunctival capillaries, as well as through the nasal mucosa, the oropharynx, and the gastrointestinal tract after passage through the lacrimal drainage system. Absorption may be reduced by applying pressure on the nasal canthus, thereby occluding the puncta and preventing entry into the lacrimal drainage system and thus the gastrointestinal tract. Although the actual blood levels obtained as a result of eye drops usually are low, sensitive individuals or those with compromised body systems (congestive heart failure, emphysema, senile dementia) most often develop complications.

a. Cardiopulmonary decompensation: Timolol maleate is a nonspecific beta blocker used to reduce intraocular tension. Precipitation of acute asthmatic attacks in asymptomatic patients have been reported.[13, 14] We have seen two cases of bronchospasm precipitated in patients with preexisting obstructive pulmonary disease. Timolol has also been associated with precipitating congestive heart failure in a patient with rheumatic heart disease.[15] Bradycardia and syncope have been reported,[14] as well as the aggravation of myasthenia gravis.[16] Epinephrine and 10 per cent phenylephrine drops have been linked to complications of excessive beta stimulation, such as severe hypertensive reactions, myocardial infarctions, and coronary artery spasm.[17, 18]

b. Effects of anticholinesterase agents: Anticholinesterase agents, such as echothiophate iodide and demecarium bromide, used to treat primary open angle glaucoma, cause depression of true cholinesterase and pseudocholinesterase. Although the usual effects might be abdominal cramps, diarrhea, sweating, and weakness, an episode of cardiac arrest[19] and refractory bronchospasm[20] have been reported. Most important in preoperative evaluation, the inhibition of pseudocholinesterase may prevent the breakdown of succinylcholine, leading to prolonged apnea. It is critically important that the consulting physician convey to the anesthesiologist the fact that the patient is using anticholinesterase agents.

c. Effects in central nervous system: Both scopolamine and atropine can cause confusion, excitement, and hallucinations in children, as well as the elderly.[22, 23, 24] When called to evaluate an elderly patient with a new onset of confusion or hallucinations after ocular surgery, one should review the drops carefully to see whether either of these agents is being used.

The systemic manifestations of eye drops have been well documented. The occasional serious complications most often occur in patients with compromised cardiopulmonary or CNS function. When taking the medical history from these patients, the drops should be reviewed along with the systemic medications. By remembering the systemic effects of eye drops, one may prevent serious complications in some cases and, in others, find that perplexing problems have simple solutions.

## REFERENCES

1. Duncalf D, Gartner S, Carol B: Mortality in association with ophthalmic surgery. Am J Ophthalmol 69:610, 1970.
2. Kincaid WH (ed): Deaths in hospitals following surgery. Ann Arbor Commission on Professional and Hospital Activities 9:1, 1971.
3. Quigley HA: Mortality associated with ophthalmic surgery: A twenty-year experience at the Wilmer Institute. Am J Ophthalmol 77:517, 1974.
4. Petruscak J, Smith B, Breslin P: Mortality related to ophthalmological surgery. Arch Ophthalmol 89:106, 1973.
5. Kaplan NR, Reba RC: Pulmonary embolism as the leading cause of ophthalmologic surgery mortality. Am J Ophthalmol 73:159, 1972.
6. Wolf GL, Seamus L, Berlin I: Intraocular surgery with general anesthesia. Arch Ophthalmol 93:323, 1975.
7. Backer BA, Tinker JH, Robertson DM, Vlietrstra RE: Myocardial reinfarction following local anesthesia for ophthalmic surgery. Anesth Analg 59:257,1980.
8. Steen PA, Tinker JH, Tarhan S: Myocardial reinfarction after anesthesia and surgery. JAMA 239:2566, 1978.
9. Goldman L, Caldera DL: Risks of general anesthesia and elective operations in the hypertensive patient. Anesthesiology 50:285, 1979.
10. Hall DL, Steen WH, Drummond JW: Anticoagulants and cataract surgery. Ann Ophthalmol 12:759, 1980.
11. Adler AG, McElwain GE, Merli GJ, Martin JH: Systemic affects of eye drops. Arch Intern Med 142:2293, 1982.
12. Jeglum EL: Ocular therapeutic. Nurs Clin North Am 16:453, 1981.
13. Charan NB, Lakshminarayan S: Pulmonary affects of topical timolol. Arch Intern Med 140:843, 1980.
14. McMahon CD, Shaffer RN, Hoskins HD, et al.: Adverse affects experienced by patients taking timolol. Am J Ophthalmol 88:736, 1979.
15. Britman NA: Cardiac affects of topical timolol. N Engl J Med 300:562, 1979.
16. Kohn A: Systemic affects of timolol. JAMA 243:1131, 1980.
17. Fraunfelder FT, Scafidi AF: Possible affects from topical ocular 10% phenylephrine. Am J Ophthalmol 85:447, 1978.
18. Adler AG, McElwain GE, Martin JH, Jeglum EL: Coronary artery spasm induced by phenylephrine eye drops. Arch Intern Med 191:1384, 1981.
19. Humphreys JA, Holmes JH: Systemic affects produced by echothiophate iodide in treatment of glaucoma. Arch Ophthalmol 69:737, 1963.
20. Fratto C: Provocation of bronchospasm by eye drops. Ann Intern Med 88:362, 1978.
21. Johnson PD: Period of prolonged apnea following suxamethonium chloride. Br J Anaesth 26:427, 1954.
22. Hoefnagel D: Toxic affects of atropine and homatoprine eye drops in children. N Engl J Med 264:168, 1961.

23. Freund M, Meun S: Toxic affects of scopolamine eye drops. Am J
    Ophthalmol *70*:637, 1970.
24. Carpenter WT Jr: Precipitous mental deterioration following cyclo-
    plegia with 0.2% cyclopentolate HCl. Arch Ophthalmol *78*:445,
    1967.

## VI.  THE PREGNANT PATIENT

# CHOLECYSTECTOMY

### A.  PREOPERATIVE EVALUATION

1. Background and purpose

   The incidence of cholelithiasis in the United States, as
   shown by autopsy studies, is about 20 per cent in females
   and 8 per cent in males. Of these, 50 per cent will
   experience symptoms of biliary colic or acute cholecystitis. Thus, women have a higher incidence of calculus
   formation and are at greater risk of developing biliary
   disease. Nilsson showed that during the menstrual years,
   women have a higher incidence of gallbladder disease
   and therefore an increased potential to complicate pregnancy by this process.[1] With this in mind, the internist
   can aid his or her ob/gyn colleagues in the management
   of a pregnant female with acute cholecystitis.

2. Clinical assessment

   a. The incidence of cholecystectomy in pregnancy has
      been shown in four studies (Table 13–12).

   b. The second trimester is the optimal time for surgery,
      since the peak period for spontaneous abortion has
      passed and the uterus is not large enough to impinge
      on the operating field.[4]

   c. In uncomplicated cholecystitis, there is no increase in
      maternal mortality, and fetal loss approximates 5 per
      cent.[6]

   d. If pancreatitis complicates cholelithiasis, maternal
      mortality increases to 15 per cent and fetal loss
      approaches 60 per cent.[5, 6]

**TABLE 13–12. Incidence of Cholecystectomy in Pregnancy**

| Study | Incidence |
| --- | --- |
| Sparkman[2] | 0.062% |
| Aufses[3] | 0.03% |
| Hill et al.[4] | 0.079% |
| Printen & Oh[5] | 0.3% |

  e. Vigorous medical management should be the first line of therapy.
  f. Laboratory studies
    (1) CBC with platelets
    (2) Electrolytes, BUN, and glucose
    (3) SGOT, SGPT, alkaline phosphatate, bilirubin
    (4) Amylase
    (5) Prothrombin time and partial thromboplastin time
    (6) Urinalysis
    (7) ECG
    (8) Ultrasound of gallbladder if possible
3. Perioperative management
  1. Prophylaxis:[8] The following patients undergoing elective surgery should receive antibiotic prophylaxis:
    a. Previous biliary tract surgery
    b. Obstructive jaundice
    c. Common bile duct obstruction with jaundice

    } Cefazolin 1 gm IM on call to the operating room, or IV with induction of anesthesia

  b. Prophylaxis for endocarditis: See Chapter 2.

## REFERENCES

1. Nilsson S: Gallbladder disease and sex hormones: A statistical study. Acta Chir Scand *132*:275, 1966.
2. Sparkman RS: Gallstones in young women. Ann Surg 45:813, 1957.
3. Aufses AH Jr: Biliary tract disease, Medical, Surgical, and Gynecological Complications of Pregnancy, ed 2, Rovinsky JJ, Guttenmacher AF (eds). Baltimore, Williams & Wilkins, 1965, p. 251.
4. Hill LM, Johnson CE, Lee RA: Cholecystectomy in pregnancy. Obstet Gynecol *46*:291, 1975.
5. Printen JJ, Oh RA: Cholecystectomy during pregnancy. Am J Surg *44*:432, 1978.
6. Naunyn B, Schroder H: Acute cholecystitis in pregnancy and the puerperium. Am J Surg *38*:314, 1972.
7. Kammerer WS: Nonobstetric surgery during pregnancy. Med Clin North Am *63*:1157, 1979.
8. Antimicrobial prophylaxis for surgery. The Medical Letter *23*:77, 1981.

# APPENDECTOMY

## A. PREOPERATIVE EVALUATION

  1. Background and purpose
     Appendicitis can occur at any stage during pregnancy.

The incidence of this complicating factor varies from 1 in 355[1] to 1 in 11,479.[2] Symptoms and signs vary according to the stage of pregnancy and make differential diagnosis difficult. The internist who is requested to evaluate the patient preoperatively will be concerned with appropriate diagnosis and with safety of mother and fetus with respect to medication.

2. Clinical assessment
   a. Incidence: Studies concerning the incidence of appendicitis in pregnancy are listed in Table 13–13.
   b. Anatomy: Figure 13–4 depicts the migration of the appendix during various months of the pregnancy.
   c. Fetus: When the appendix has perforated and peritonitis is present, fetal mortality is 35.7 per cent.[3] If the appendix has not perforated, the mortality is 1.5 per cent.[3]
   d. Mother: Black,[1] in a review of 373 cases, showed no maternal deaths in the first trimester, but maternal mortality was 3.9 per cent in the second trimester, 10 per cent in the third, and 16.7 per cent intrapartum.
   e. Laboratory studies
      (1) CBC with platelets
      (2) Electrolytes, BUN, and glucose
      (3) Prothrombin time and partial thromboplastin time
      (4) Urinalysis

**TABLE 13–13. Incidence of Appendicitis During Pregnancy in 503,496 Deliveries**

| Authors | No. of Cases | No. of Deliveries | Incidence |
|---|---|---|---|
| Cunningham et al, 1975 | 34 | 91,800 | 1/2700 |
| Finch et al, 1974 | 56 | 94,000 | 1/1678 |
| Kurtz et al, 1964 | 41 | 84,260 | 1/2059 |
| Lee et al, 1965 | 20 | 16,100 | 1/805 |
| Mohammed et al, 1975 | 20 | 34,270 | 1/1713 |
| O'Neill, 1969 | 62 | 91,500 | 1/1476 |
| Sarson et al, 1963 | 11 | 11,000 | 1/1000 |
| Taylor, 1972 | 55 | 38,719 | 1/705 |
| Thomford et al, 1969 | 22 | 22,000 | 1/1000 |
| Present series | 12 | 25,847 | 1/2154 |
| Total | 333 | 503,496 | 1/1500 |

From Babaknia A, Hossein P, Woodruff WD: Appendicitis during pregnancy. Obstet Gynecol 50:40, 1977.

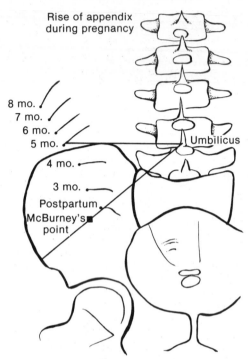

**Figure 13–4.** Changes in position and direction of appendix during pregnancy. After the fifth month of pregnancy the appendix lies at the crest level and rises above this level during the last trimester. The postpartum position of the appendix corresponds to its position in the nonpregnant state. Roentgenologically, the base of the appendix is usually found medial to McBurney's point. The average position of the umbilicus corresponds to the point at which a line extended horizontally from the iliac crest crosses the spine. (Reprinted with permission from Baer et al: Appendicitis in pregnancy with changes in position and axis of normal appendix in pregnancy. JAMA 98:1359, 1932.)

## B. PERIOPERATIVE MANAGEMENT

1. Prophylaxis:[4]

Clindamycin 600 mg IM or IV
*or*
Doxycycline 200 mg IV          30 minutes to 1 hour be-
*or*                          fore procedure
Cefoxitin 1 gm IV

2. Endocarditis prophylaxis: See Chapter 2.
3. Therapeutic: When fever and leukocytosis are present the following regimens can be used:
   a. Aminoglycoside 1.5 mg/kg/q8h IM or IV plus clindamycin 600 mg IV q6h
   b. Aminoglycoside 1.5 mg/kg/q8h IM or IV plus cefoxitin 1 gm q6h

## REFERENCES

1. Black WP: Acute appendicitis in pregnancy. Br Med J *1*:1938, 1960.
2. Tedenat J. Appendicite chez la femma enceinte. Bull Soc d' Obstet Gynecol *14*:237, 1925.
3. Babaknia A, Hossein P, Woodruff JD: Appendicitis during pregnancy. Obstet Gynecol *50*:40, 1977.
4. Hirschmann JV: Rational antibiotic prophylaxis. Hosp Pract *16*:105–109, 113–120, 123, 1982.

# MYASTHENIA GRAVIS

## A. PREOPERATIVE EVALUATION

1. Background and purpose
   Myasthenia gravis occurs in all ages and is more common in females than in males. The peak incidence is in the third decade for females, and in 20 per cent onset is before age twenty-one. This is an important consideration, since these are the childbearing years for women. The consultant is mainly concerned with maintenance of therapy and the necessary alterations for labor and delivery.
2. Clinical assessment
   a. Pregnancy
      (1) The course of myasthenia gravis is highly variable and unpredictable. When exacerbations occur, they are most likely in the first trimester or in the postpartum period.[1, 2]
      (2) The course during a previous pregnancy does not indicate what course the disease might take in future pregnancies.[3]
      (3) Induced abortion does not alter the course of the disease, and exacerbation of symptoms is not an indication for termination of pregnancy.[4]
      (4) Use of anticholinesterase drug in pregnancy has been associated with a higher incidence of spon-

TABLE 13–14. Therapeutic Regimen for Myasthenia Gravis
During Pregnancy

| Drug | Route | Frequency |
|------|-------|-----------|
| Pyridostigmine bromide (Mestinon) | PO 60 mg (liquid 5 ml = 60 mg; IM or IV = 2 mg) | q4–6h |
| Pyridostigmine bromide time spansules (Mestinon/Time Span.) | PO 180 mg | q12h |
| Neostigmine bromide (Prostigmin) | PO 15 mg | q4–6h |
| Neostigmine methylsulfate (Prostigmin Injectable) | 0.5 mg IM or IV | q4–6h |
| Ambenonium chloride (Mytelase) | PO 30 mg | q4–6h |

taneous abortion and premature labor, as reported by Osserman.[5] A study by Plauche did not demonstrate an increased incidence.[1]

## B. PERIOPERATIVE MANAGEMENT

1. Dosage of anticholinesterases (Table 13–19)
   a. Anticholinesterase therapy must be maintained during labor, and the drugs should be given IM.[6]
   b. Because the first ten days postpartum are critical, anticholinesterases should be restarted as soon as possible.
   c. Make sure preoperative sedation is minimal.
   d. Breast feeding is not a contraindication, because anticholinesterases are not transmitted into breast milk.
2. Labor and delivery
   a. Myasthenia gravis is not an indication for cesarean section.
   b. In patients witih preeclampsia, the use of magnesium sulfate may precipitate muscle weakness and respiratory insufficiency. This drug is contraindicated in patients with myasthenia gravis.[7]
3. Postpartum
   Plauche reported that 57 per cent of patients had exacerbation of symptoms and that 2.4 per cent died from myasthenic crises during the first ten days postpartum.[1]

## REFERENCES

1. Plauche WC: Myasthenia gravis in pregnancy. Am J Obstet Gynecol 88:404–409, 1964.
2. Simpson JA: Myasthenia gravis: A new hypothesis. Scott Med J 5:419–436, 1960.
3. Kosovsky N, Spurt H, Osserman KE: Pregnancy in myasthenia gravis. Am J Med 19:718–720, 1955.
4. Hay DM: Myasthenia gravis and pregnancy. J Obstet Gynaec Brit Comm. 76:323–329, 1969.
5. Osserman KE: Obstetrics in myasthenia gravis, Osserman KE (ed). New York, Grune and Stratton, 1958, pp 239–242.
6. Rolbin SH, Levinson G, Shnider SM, Wright RG: Anesthetic considerations for myasthenia gravis and pregnancy. Anesth Analg 57:441, 1978.
7. Cohen BA, London RS, Goldstein PJ: Myasthenia gravis and pre-eclampsia. Obstet Gynecol 48(Suppl):355–375, 1975.

## VII. THE PSYCHIATRIC PATIENT

### A. PREOPERATIVE EVALUATION

1. Background and purpose

An estimated 10 per cent of patients visiting an internist have a psychiatric disorder, most often a neurosis.[1] The prevalence of psychotropic drug use, especially benzodiazepines, as well as alcohol and drug abuse is also of concern. A number of these patients are elderly and frequently have an underlying disease. The most critical factors in assessing psychiatric patients in the preoperative period are definition of underlying illness and careful assessment of drug use and potential adverse interactions.

The major psychiatric illnesses that may be confused with organic disease, specifically neurosis, acute psychosis, and the affective disorders, are outlined in this chapter. In addition, the problem of drug dependence is reviewed. Alcohol abuse and withdrawal are dealt with elsewhere in the text. Emphasis is placed on differential diagnosis, acute therapy, and management through the perioperative period. Major psychotropic drug side effects and interactions are discussed, as well as postoperative delirium and evaluation of the patient for electroconvulsive therapy.

2. Clinical assessment

A great deal of information regarding the patient's psychological state may be obtained during history taking. Important areas to stress are previous psychiatric history, previous surgical and anesthestic history, medication usage—both psychotropic and nonpsychotropic—and presence of other illness. A thorough physical examination is essential, with attention to the mental status examination.[2] Laboratory studies of interest are discussed within the specific topics.

3. Risk factors

Psychiatric illness itself is rarely a significant risk factor for surgery,[3] although severe illness may make management more difficult. Therefore, the major factors affecting risk are as follows:

   a. Presence and degree of other medical illness
   b. Significant depression with severe vegetative signs
   c. Severe agitation
   d. Acute intoxication
   e. Use of tricyclic or tetracyclic antidepressants in patients with cardiac disease or use of monoamine oxidase inhibitors

## B. SPECIFIC ENTITIES

1. Neurosis

   a. Signs and symptoms: The neuroses comprise a number of disorders, including phobia, panic disorders, anxiety states, hysteria, psychosexual disorders, and hypochondriasis. Although an exact definition for psychosis is difficult, it can be viewed as one end of a spectrum of dysfunction with neurosis at the other end. Within this framework the key point is the patient's ability to test reality. The neurotic patient most often can function socially and has minimal impairment of personality, unlike the psychotic patient, who often has marked distortion of the personality with severe abnormalities in social function.[1]

   All neuroses are marked by an abnormality in behavior. The neuroses of most interest to the medical consultant are those that mimic acute or chronic organic disease. The most common of these neuroses are anxiety states, including panic and general anxiety disorders, somatoform or hysterical disorders, and conversion disorders. The symptoms of panic and general anxiety disorders are listed in Table 13–15. As can be seen, they are predominantly autonomic or cardiovascular in origin. Many of the same symptoms are present in hysteria (Table 13–16). The conversion disorders frequently have symptoms of paralysis, blindness, sensory abnormalities, aphasia, amnesia, urinary retention, and tics, without demonstrable anatomic or physiologic changes.

**TABLE 13–15. Symptoms of Anxiety Neurosis**

| Symptoms | 60 Patients (%) | 102 Controls* (%) |
|---|---|---|
| Palpitation | 97 | 9 |
| Tires easily | 93 | 19 |
| Breathlessness | 90 | 13 |
| Nervousness | 88 | 27 |
| Chest pain | 85 | 10 |
| Sighing | 79 | 16 |
| Dizziness | 78 | 16 |
| Faintness | 70 | 12 |
| Apprehensiveness | 61 | 3 |
| Headache | 58 | 26 |
| Paresthesias | 58 | 7 |
| Weakness | 56 | 3 |
| Trembling | 54 | 17 |
| Breath unsatisfactory | 53 | 4 |
| Insomnia | 53 | 4 |
| Unhappiness | 50 | 2 |
| Shakiness | 47 | 16 |
| Fatigued all the time | 45 | 6 |
| Sweating | 42 | 33 |
| Fear of death | 42 | 2 |
| Smothering | 40 | 3 |
| Syncope | 37 | 11 |
| Nervous chill | 24 | 0 |
| Urinary frequency | 18 | 2 |
| Vomiting and diarrhea | 14 | 0 |
| Anorexia | 12 | 3 |
| Paralysis | 0 | 0 |
| Blindness | 0 | 0 |

*Healthy controls consisted of 550 mean and 11 women from a large industrial plant, and 41 healthy postpartum women from the Boston Lying-In Hospital. From Wheeler EO, White PD, Reed EW, Cohen ME: Neurocirculatory asthenia (anxiety neurosis, effort syndrome, neurasthenia). JAMA *142*:878–889, 1950.

In most cases the diagnosis of neurosis is fairly straightforward, but in instances of acute panic attacks and anxiety states, as well as in a number of hysterical and conversion disorders, a distinction must be made between a psychiatric illness and an organic illness. Thyrotoxicosis may mimic acute panic or anxiety, but such findings as lack of eye signs, normal heart rate during sleep, and lack of goiter and normal serum thyroxine can be helpful in excluding this condition. Mitral valve prolapse (MVP) frequently is associated with these disorders; therefore, a clear-cut distinction

**TABLE 13–16. Frequency of Symptoms in Hysteria**

| Symptom | % | Symptom | % | Symptom | % |
|---|---|---|---|---|---|
| Dyspnea | 72 | Weight loss | 28 | Back pain | 88 |
| Palpitation | 60 | Anorexia | 60 | Joint pain | 84 |
| Chest pain | 72 | Nausea | 80 | Extremity pain | 84 |
| Dizziness | 84 | Vomiting | 32 | Burning pains in rectum, vagina, mouth | 28 |
| Headache | 80 | Abdominal pain | 80 | Other bodily pain | 36 |
| Anxiety attacks | 64 | Abdominal bloating | 68 | Depressed feelings | 64 |
| Fatigue | 84 | Food intolerances | 48 | Phobias | 48 |
| Blindness | 20 | Diarrhea | 20 | Vomiting all nine months of pregnancy | 20 |
| Paralysis | 12 | Constipation | 64 | Nervous | 92 |
| Anesthesia | 32 | Dysuria | 44 | Had to quit working because felt bad | 44 |
| Aphonia | 44 | Urinary retention | 8 | Trouble doing anything because felt bad | 72 |
| Lump in throat | 28 | Dysmenorrhea—premarital only | 4 | Cried a lot | 60 |
| Fits or convulsions | 20 | Dysmenorrhea—prepregnancy only | 8 | Felt life was hopeless | 28 |
| Faints | 56 | Dysmenorrhea—other | 48 | Always sickly (most of life) | 40 |
| Unconsciousness | 16 | Menstrual irregularity | 48 | Thought of dying | 48 |
| Amnesia | 8 | Excessive menstrual bleeding | 48 | Wanted to die | 36 |
| Visual blurring | 64 | Sexual indifference | 44 | Thought of suicide | 28 |
| Visual hallucination | 12 | Frigidity (absence of orgasm) | 24 | Attempted suicide | 12 |
| Deafness | 4 | Dyspareunia | 52 | | |
| Olfactory hallucination | 16 | | | | |
| Weakness | 84 | | | | |
| Sudden fluctuations in weight | 16 | | | | |

From Perley MJ, Guze SB: Hysteria—the stability and usefulness of clinical criteria. N Engl J Med 266:421–426, 1962.

between the two is difficult if the auscultatory or echocardiographic finding suggests MVP. If MVP is found, antibiotic prophylaxis for endocarditis should be considered in the appropriate surgical setting (see Chapter 2). In patients taking insulin or oral hypoglycemic agents, hypoglycemia must be ruled out. Pheochromocytoma can resemble these syndromes, especially in regard to its episodic nature. A strong suspicion of this tumor requires thorough evaluation before surgery. Other diagnoses to consider are pulmonary embolus, myocardial infarction, hypoxia, and drug overdose (hallucinogens) or withdrawal (alcohol, barbiturates). Hyperventilation will frequently reproduce symptoms of acute anxiety attacks and may be a helpful diagnostic test.

Hysterical symptoms of paralysis, paresthesias, and blindness may be separated from organic symptoms quite easily in most cases by careful neurologic examination. Usually, discrepancies exist between the symptoms and the physical signs. Frequently, the symptoms have no corresponding anatomic distribution. In certain rare circumstances nerve conduction studies, electromyography, or other specialized tests may be helpful. These should be used in consultation with a neurologist.

b. Perioperative management: During an acute panic or anxiety attack careful reassurance, with or without a benzodiazepine, is often helpful. Long-term management of panic attack usually involves use of an antidepressant.[4] These disorders rarely present a significant risk for surgery if other medical conditions are excluded and the acute episode is controlled. Often a delay of one or two hours is sufficient for a patient with an anxiety or panic disorder to adjust to the need for surgery.

For the patient with an established diagnosis, the following recommendation can be made. The hospital environment should be as supportive as possible. For elective surgery, benzodiazepines should be withdrawn slowly with the help of a psychiatrist if the patient has taken them continuously for longer than four months. With use of less than four months, it is probably safe to stop the drug abruptly with only minimal withdrawal symptoms of anxiety.

In elective surgery, it is wise to discontinue tricyclics slowly over several weeks before surgery. In emergent surgery, benzodiazepines should be continued periop-eratively to avoid withdrawal phenomenon. IV or IM routes may be used. If tricyclic antidepressants cannot be stopped preoperatively, the patient should have careful ECG monitoring for arrhythmias, with the drug being restarted as soon as possible postopera-tively.

2. Psychosis

   a. Signs and symptoms: The acutely agitated patient may occasionally present in a "psychotic" state marked by inability to test reality. There is frequently overwhelm-ing suspiciousness, hallucinations, marked withdrawal from the environment, and confusion.[1] A careful search for underlying central nervous system disease, such as tumor or infection, as well as for metabolic or toxic insult should be made. This evaluation should include, in addition to a thorough physical examina-tion, CBC, arterial blood gas analysis, chest x-ray, electrolytes, serum calcium, BUN, creatinine, liver function tests, urinalysis, drug screen of blood and urine, and a CT scan of the head and lumbar puncture, if necessary.

   b. Perioperative management: If no underlying disorder can be found, treatment with a butyrophenone may be useful to control the acute episode until a more definitive psychiatric diagnosis can be established. If emergency surgery is needed, butyrophenones are the preferred agents because of their low potential for cardiovascular toxicity. IM injections of haloperidol 5 to 10 mg may be given every hour until a clinical response is achieved. Most patients show significant benefit from less than 40 mg. A failure to show any improvement should lead to reassessment of the di-agnosis. This treatment is complicated by the devel-opment of acute dystonias in up to half of all patients treated. Use of oral benztropine 1 to 2 mg twice daily may be helpful to prevent these uncomfortable side effects.[5]

      In the chronically psychotic patient on therapy it is recommended that antipsychotic medication be stopped several days before surgery. This rarely leads to an exacerbation of the psychiatric condition.[3] If it is felt that the risk of exacerbation is high, then the antipsychotic agent can be continued parenterally through the perioperative period.[6] In the presence of underlying cardiovascular disease careful attention must be given to hemodynamics and drug interactions discussed later.

3. Affective disorders
   a. Sign and symptoms: The affective disorders of importance to the preoperative consultant are unipolar depression and bipolar illness, or manic-depressive illness. The distinction is important, since psychopharmacology is different (tricyclic antidepressants and monoamine oxidase inhibitors in depression and lithium in bipolar illness). Of interest to the medical consultant is the differentiation from organic illness and the evaluation and management of drug use.[7]

   Unipolar illness is most often associated with sleepiness, insomia, appetite and weight changes, early morning wakening, and feelings of helplessness. Bipolar illness can present as depression, but about 80 per cent of the time it presents with the signs and symptoms of acute mania: pressured speech, hyperactivity, verbosity, grandiosity, irritability, and euphoria.

   Several medical problems mimic depression. Hypothyroidism is the most important of these. It usually can be excluded on the basis of physical findings and serum thyroxine ($T_4$) and thyroid-stimulating hormone (TSH) determination. Other considerations are hypoadrenalism, hypopituitarism, hypercalcemia, anemia, occult carcinoma, occult congestive heart failure, organic brain disease, electrolyte imbalance, and chronic drug or alcohol use; most of these possibilities can be eliminated by careful examination and a battery of simple laboratory tests. Drugs associated with depression are antihypertensives—including alphamethyldopa, beta blockers, clonidine, reserpine, and guanethidine—levodopa, and corticosteroids. Bipolar illness in the manic phase may superficially resemble thyrotoxicosis or acute intoxication, but differentiation on clinical grounds is rarely difficult. In patients over age 50 presenting with mania, a CNS tumor must be ruled out.

   In most patients wtih an undiagnosed severe depression, a small number of laboratory tests, in conjunction with the history and physical examination should allow the consultant to exclude most medical illnesses that might compromise the patient during surgery. Chest x-ray, ECG, CBC, $T_4$, TSH, calcium, electrolytes, BUN, creatinine, urinalysis, and drug screen are probably adequate to accomplish this. If, as noted previously, a patient over age 50 presents with mania, a CT scan of the head should be done to exclude a tumor.

b. Perioperative management: A newly diagnosed patient with depression is not at significantly increased risk for surgery unless the vegetative signs are severe. Most patients can have antidepressant medication started several days postoperatively if it is felt that drug therapy is needed. Severely depressed patients should have at least one or two months of therapy before an elective surgical procedure.[3] An attempt should be made to control the patient with bipolar illness with lithium carbonate before surgery. If urgent surgery is needed in either of these groups, it should not be withheld. Careful attention should be paid to pulmonary care and bed care for the patient with severe vegetative signs to prevent postoperative pneumonia, skin breakdown, and thromboembolic complications. The acutely manic patient can be managed with butyrophenones in a manner similar to the patient with acute psychosis. Electroconvulsive therapy may be useful for rapid control before surgery in certain patients with severe illness.[7]

In the patient with known disease the use of antidepressants should be stopped three to seven days preoperatively. This rarely results in significant worsening of depression.[3] In elderly patients or patients with cardiac disease it may be best to discontinue the antidepressant slowly, over several weeks preoperatively, to minimize withdrawal and possibly cardiac toxicity.[6] Lithium carbonate can be stopped one day preoperatively with little risk of acute mania. All medications can safely be restarted several days postoperatively.

## D. OVERVIEW OF MEDICATIONS USED TO TREAT PSYCHIATRIC ILLNESS

This section deals with individual classes of drugs. Major side effects and drug interactions are given, as well as recommendations for preoperative management of patients using these agents. A comprehensive table of drug interactions can be found in Gaultieri and Powell.[8]

1. Benzodiazepines
   a. Side effects: Sedation
   b. Drug interactions: Increases phenytoin levels, increases CNS depression of opiates and other sedatives

    c. Preoperative management
      (1) With use of low dose or for less than four months, drug can be stopped with occasional mild withdrawal symptoms (tremor, diaphoresis, nausea).
      (2) With use of high dose or for longer than four months, drug should be withdrawn slowly over one to two weeks preoperatively, preferably with consultative assistance from a psychiatrist. If this is not possible, drug should be continued perioperatively.

2. Meprobamate and barbiturates
    a. Side effects: CNS depression
    b. Drug interactions: Induces hepatic microsomal enzymes, resulting in increased metabolism of anticoagulants, analgesics, and some antibiotics
    c. Preoperative management: If use is of short duration (less than three months), the medication can be stopped. If use is of long duration, these medications should be withdrawn slowly preoperatively (as with benzodiazepines) or continued if there is no time to withdraw the patient.

3. Tricyclic and tetracyclic antidepressants
    a. Side effects: Sedation, urinary retention, dry mouth, glaucoma, blurred vision, confusion, weight gain, postural hypotension, cardiac effects (including T wave changes, intraventricular conduction delays, atrial and ventricular arrhythmias, and heart failure—all usually only at toxic blood levels), elevated hepatic enzymes, agranulocytosis, parkinsonism, and seizures[9]
    b. Drug interactions: See Table 13–17.
    c. Preoperative management: In patients with no underlying disease it is probably safe to stop the medication several days preoperatively, although the patient may experience a mild withdrawal syndrome of chills, malaise, and muscle aches. In the elderly patient or the patient with cardiac disease it would be best to taper the agent slowly, over several weeks preoperatively. If urgent surgery is needed, patient should be monitored carefully for arrhythmias and heart failure.

4. Monoamine oxidase inhibitors
    a. Side effects: Transient anticholinergic effects, hypertensive crises with foods containing tyramine (cheeses, red wines, etc., although these are probably uncommon with reasonable dietary compliance)[10]
    b. Drug interactions:
      (1) Inhibit hepatic enzymes, leading to decreased metabolism of sedatives and narcotics

**TABLE 13–17. Drug Interactions**

| Type of Drug | When Combined With | Produce These Effects |
|---|---|---|
| Tricyclic agents | Monoamine oxidase inhibitors | Hyperpyrexia, convulsions |
| | Thyroxin | Increased antidepressant effect |
| | Alcohol | Decreased antidepressant effect |
| | | Marked sedation, respiratory depression, learning problem |
| | Methylphenidate (Ritalin) | Increased antidepressant effect—brief deviation |
| | Barbiturates | Decreased antidepressant effect |
| | Antiparkinsonian drugs | Additive anticholinergic effect |
| | Oral contraceptives | Decreased antidepressant effect |
| | Epinephrine | Hypertensive crisis by inhibition of norepinephrine reuptake |
| | Dicumarol | Increased anticoagulant effect |
| | Chlorothiazide (Diuril) | Increased hypotensive effect |
| | Phenothiazines | Increased antidepressant effect to a point, then decreased effect |
| | Guanethidine (Ismelin) | Decreased antihypertensive effect |
| | Clonidine (Catapres) | Decreased antidepressant effect |
| | Methyldopa (Aldomet) | Decreased antidepressive effect |
| | Propranolol (Inderal) | Decreased antidepressive effect |

| Monoamine oxidase inhibitors | Tricyclic antidepressants | Hypertensive crisis |
| | Antidiabetic agents | Increased hypoglycemia |
| | Levodopa | Hypertensive crisis |
| | Meperidine | Hypertension, convulsions, coma by alternate metabolic pathway to normeperidine |
| | Epinephrine | Hypertensive crisis |
| | Methylphenidate | Hypertensive crisis |
| | Tyramine in foods and beverages | Hypertensive crisis by increased norepinephrine release |
| | Amphetamines | Hypertensive crisis |
| | Central nervous system depressants | Increased depressant effect |
| | Antiparkinsonian drugs | Increased anticholinergic effects |

From Rosenbaum AH, Maruta T, Richelson E: Drugs that alter mood. I: Tricyclic agents and monoamine oxidase inhibitors. Mayo Clin Proc 54:341, 1979.

(2) Inhibitor of monoamine oxidase, causing sympathomimetic crises with such agents as tyramine, levodopa, antihistamines, sympathomimetics, amphetamines, and tricyclic antidepressants. They may increase the neuromuscular blockage produced by succinylcholine (also see Table 13–17).[11]

c. Preoperative management: These drugs should be stopped several weeks preoperatively for elective surgery. For emergent surgery, continuous intra-arterial pressure monitoring and cardiac monitoring should be done with avoidance, if possible, of sympathomimetic drugs. Treatment of sympathetic crises should be managed in a fashion similar to pheochromocytoma.

5. Lithium
   a. Side effects: GI distress, tremor, drowsiness; toxic symptoms: nausea, vomiting, cogwheel rigidity, edema, weight gain, unsteady gait, muscle twitching, slurred speech, hypothyroidism, polyuria, nephrogenic diabetes insipidius, seizures, coma;[12] T wave inversions and QRS widening can be observed on the ECG.[13]
   b. Drug interactions: Diuretics (except osmotic agents and acetazolamide) decrease renal excretion of lithium. Phenothiazines increase lithium toxicity and lithium potentiates the cardiovascular effects of tricyclic antidepressants. Lithium can also prolong the effect of neuromuscular blocking agents (see Table 13–18).[12]
   c. Preoperative evaluation: BUN or creatinine, electrolytes, and serum lithium levels should be measured and an ECG obtained. For elective surgery, the drug should be discontinued one day preoperatively. For emergent surgery, a nontoxic patient has little increase in risk, although neuromuscular blocking agents and diuretics must be used with caution. If toxicity is present (lithium level greater than 2), it can be managed by discontinuation of the drug, gastric suction (lithium is secreted into the stomach), sodium chloride infusion, and administration of mannitol and aminophylline to decrease proximal renal tubular reabsorption of lithium.

6. Neuroleptic agents
   a. Side effects: The phenothiazines and butyrophenones can cause a variety of side effects, with different agents in each class manifesting these effects to different degrees. The most common side effects are postural hypotension, anticholinergic effects (dry mouth, blurred vision, tachycardia), and extrapyramidal ef-

**TABLE 13–18. Antidepressant and Antimanic Drugs**

| Drug Class | Examples | When Combined With | Produce These Effects |
|---|---|---|---|
| | | Haloperidol (Haldol) | Increase in haloperidol toxicity |
| | | Tricyclic antidepressants | Increase in depression with toxiciy |
| | | | Additive antidepressant effect |
| | | | Decrease in blood pressure if the dosage is too high; delirium and seizures |
| | | | Increase in blood pressure if hypotension is secondary to tricyclic agents |
| Lithium carbonate | Eskalith Lithane Lithonate | Methyldopa (Aldomet) | Increase in lithium toxicity; resembles Parkinson's disease |
| | | Sodium-depleting diuretics | Increase in lithium toxicity |
| | | Phenothiazines | Increase in phenothiazine toxicity |
| | | | Increase in depression with toxicity |
| | | Diazepam (Valium), oxazepam (Serax) | Increase in depression |
| | | Neuromuscular blocking agents | Potentiation of blockade |

From Rosenbaum AH, Maruta T, Richelson E: Drugs that alter mood. II: Lithium. Mayo Clin Prac 54:405, 1979.

fects (Parkinsonlike syndrome, tardive dyskinesia, and acute dystonia). ECG changes include PR and QT interval prolongation, widening of the QRS complex, ST segment depression, U waves, occasional premature ventricular contractions, supraventricular and ventricular tachycardia, and, rarely, ventricular fibrillation.[14]

b. Drug interactions: The CNS depressant action of alcohol, anxiolytic agents, barbiturates, and narcotics is increased by these agents. Phenothiazines also enhance the action of amphetamines, anticholinergics, and most antihypertensives. They inhibit the effect of levodopa and the antidepressant effect of MAO inhibitors but may increase the hypotensive effect of the MAO inhibitors.[11]

c. Preoperative evaluation: As mentioned earlier, the patient on antipsychotics can most often have these agents discontinued one or two days preoperatively for elective surgery without danger of acute exacerbation of illness. If the risk of exacerbation is felt to be high, the agents can be continued parenterally. Care must be taken in the use of narcotics, pressor amines, anticholinergics, and antihypertensives, as phenothiazines potentiate the actions of these drugs. A preoperative ECG and intraoperative ECG monitoring are essential. In a patient considered for neurosurgery, prophylactic anticonvulsants should be given, since phenothiazines lower the seizure threshold.

## E. DRUG DEPENDENCE

Drug dependence is of major concern to all who care for the surgical patient. The demanding behavior of this type of patient may make management difficult. In regard to the evaluation of risk, it is helpful to know the quantity of substance used, but this is usually difficult to determine.

If a patient has been using more than 0.6 gm of pentobarbital or its equivalent, he should have the medication continued through the perioperative period, with gradual withdrawal attempted postoperatively, when the patient is stable. This usuallly is best accomplished with help from a psychiatrist. Patients who abuse other sedatives and hypnotics should be managed in a similiar fashion.

Patients who are dependent on opiates should have methadone substituted during the perioperative period, with prompt referral to a methadone clinic before discharge. Amphetamine use may result in a toxic syndrome of hallucinations and overactivity. Withdrawal symptoms are fatigue, lethargy, and depression; no specific treatment is needed perioperatively. Hallucinogenic drugs may heighten preoperative anxiety, but withdrawal from them has no major adverse physiologic consequences. Alcohol dependence is discussed elsewhere in this manual.

## F. POSTOPERATIVE DELIRIUM

Postoperative syndromes can be seen in various forms. One of the most common and most alarming is acute delirium manifested by confusion, paranoia, disorientation, hallucinations, and agitation. It is important to exclude organic causes that can precipitate or aggravate this state. Common disorders include fluid, electrolyte, and acid-base disorders; hypoxia; hypoglycemia; infection; renal or hepatic failure; thyroid disease; adrenal insufficiency; hemorrhage; shock; pulmonary embolism; myocardial infarction; and drug withdrawal or toxicity. In addition to a careful review of perioperative events (anesthesia, hypotension, pain medications, etc.) and a thorough physical examination, various laboratory tests, including CBC, electrolytes, arterial blood gas analysis, renal and hepatic function tests, ECG, chest x-ray, serum glucose and calcium, may be helpful in uncovering an etiology. If focal neurologic findings are found, or if meningitis is suspected, a CT scan of the head and lumbar puncture should be performed. If all studies are negative, the etiology may be presumed to be functional, and the patient managed with careful reassurance and a supportive environment, including sensory stimulation, such as lights at night, television and radio, and frequent visits by family and friends. The use of small doses of phenothiazines or butyrophenones may also be helpful. If the delirium state continues, serial reassessment of the previously mentioned parameters needs to be done to search for underlying causes.

## G. ELECTROCONVULSIVE THERAPY

Electroconvulsive therapy (ECT) has been shown to be of value in various illnesses, including severe depression, mania, and catatonia. The procedure consists of sedating the patient (usually with a short-acting barbiturate). Succinylcholine is then administered and the electrodes are applied. After ECT the patient is placed semiprone and respirations are monitored until the patient is awake. Endotracheal intubation is not done routinely.[15] This procedure is not without risk, especially for the patient with underlying cardiac, pulmonary, central nervous system, hypertensive, or musculoskeletal disorders.

In the evaluation of patients for ECT these areas are of concern to the medical consultant:

1. Use of neuromuscular blocking agents
2. The ECT episode itself
3. Effects of concomitant drug therapy

It is important in the history to define underlying medical problems and current drug use. Previous experience with anesthesia, especially neuromuscular blocking agents, is important information. The physical examination should be directed to the assessment of hypertension and cardiopulmonary disease, especially uncontrolled hypertension, congestive heart failure, severe obstructive pulmonary disease, cardiac arrhythmias, and states predisposing to hyperkalemia (renal failure, burns, crush injuries), all of which are relative contraindications to ECT. Laboratory assessment of pseudocholinesterase activity should be done.[7] Because ECT should occur without generalized convulsive activity, the pseudocholinesterase level should help to select those patients who will convulse (increased activity) and those who may have prolonged neuromuscular blockade and apnea (decreased activity).

Anticholinergic premedication is useful to prevent severe bradycardia and asystole after ECT. Atropine 0.5 to 1 mg IV is recommended just before the procedure. Continuous ECG monitoring should be carried out in all high-risk patients. Patients with pacemakers pose no special problem. The pacemaker should be in the demand mode, and atropine premedication is not needed. Care must be taken to prevent faulty grounds, which may interfere with pacemaker function.

Benzodiazepines may increase the seizure threshold and result in ineffective therapy; they should be discontinued, as outlined previously, before the procedure. MAO inhibitors should be stopped at least one week before ECT, as they can prolong the effects of sedative drugs by inhibiting hepatic enzymes, as well as rendering patients more sensitive to adrenergic stimulation. Lithium can prolong the paralytic effect of succinylcholine and potentiate the seizure activity, confusion, and memory loss that accompany ECT. Lithium should be stopped as far in advance as possible. If this is not possible, serial levels should be followed and previously outlined procedures followed to increase lithium excretion.

## REFERENCES

1. Kolb LC, Brodie HKH: The Neuroses, in Kolb LC: Modern Clinical Psychiatry, 10th ed. Philadelphia, WB Saunders, 1982, p 468.

2. Anderson WH: The physical examination in office practice. Am J Psychiatry *137*:1188, 1980.
3. Kelly MJ, Reich P: Psychiatric preparation of the surgical patient, in Vandam LD (ed): To make the Patient Ready for Anesthesia: Medical Care of the Surgical Patient. Menlo Park, California, Addison-Wesley, 1980, p 218.
4. Strain JJ, Liebowitz MR, Klein DF: Anxiety and panic attacks in the medically ill. Psychiatr Clin North Am 4:344, 1981.
5. Anderson WH, Kuehnle JC: Current concepts in psychiatry, diagnosis and early management of acute psychosis. N Engl J Med *305*:1128, 1981.
6. Blacher RS, Molitch ME: Psychiatry, in Molitch ME (ed): Management of Medical Problems in Surgical Patients. Philadelphia, FA Davis, 1982, p 425.
7. Bidder TG: Electroconvulsive therapy in the medically ill patient. Psychiatr Clin North Am *4*:391, 1981.
8. Gaultieri CT, Powell SF: Psychoactive drug interactions. Clin Psychiatry *39*:720, 1978.
9. Rosenbaum AH, Maruta T, Richelson E: Drugs that alter mood. I. Tricyclic agents and monoamine oxidase inhibitors. Mayo Clin Proc *54*:335, 1979.
10. Tollefson GD: Monoamine oxidase inhibitors: A review. J Clin Psychiatry *44*:280, 1983.
11. Marco LA, Randels PM, Sexauer JD: A guide to drug interactions with psychotropic agents. Drug Therapy *9*:45–56, 1979.
12. Rosenbaum AH, Maruta T, Richelson E: Drugs that alter mood. II. Lithium. Mayo Clin Proc *54*:401, 1979.
13. Havdala HS, Borison RL, Diamond BI: Potential hazards and applications of lithium in anesthesiology. Anesthesiology *50*:534, 1979.
14. Fowler NO, et al: Electrocardiographic changes and cardiac arrhythmias in patients receiving psychotropic drugs. Am J Cardiol *37*:223, 1976.
15. Fraser M: ECT: A Clinical Guide. New York, Wiley, 1982, p 102.

# VIII. ALCOHOL WITHDRAWAL

## A. PREOPERATIVE EVALUATION

1. Background and purpose

Alcoholism is a common problem in the United States. Identifying alcoholic patients preoperatively is important, since it allows a formulated three-point plan of management. First, a thorough history and physical examination are essential to identify other concomitant drug usage. Second, pay particular attention to (1) time and severity of signs and symptoms of withdrawal, (2) history of previous withdrawal reactions and seizures,(3) presence of concurrent medical problems that may exacerbate the severity of withdrawal.[1] And third, a rational drug protocol is designed to treat the patient and prevent the progression of symptoms. Most important to the internist is the fact that the objective is to manage the patient *up to* and *after* surgery.

2. Clinical assessment

   a. Signs and symptoms:[1, 2] The signs and symptoms of alcohol withdrawal syndrome are shown in Table 13–19 and its accompanying graph.

   b. Delirium tremens:[3, 4, 5] This occurs in 5 per cent of patients who are hospitalized for alcohol withdrawal and carries a mortality of between 10 per cent and 15 per cent. It is characterized by extreme autonomic hyperactivity (tremors, tachycardia, diaphoresis, fever, anxiety, insomnia), perceptual disorders (illusions and hallucinations), and global confusion.

   c. Seizures:[6, 7, 8, 9] Seizures occurring during withdrawal reactions are typically major motor. They occur in 41 per cent of patients between 30 and 48 hours after cessation of drinking. Only 3 per cent of patients experience status epilepticus, and this should suggest the concomitant use of short-acting sedatives by the patient or an intracranial lesion. Wolfe and Victor[9] identified the pathogenesis of seizure as resulting from alkalosis and hypomagnesemia. Seizures require treatment if they are repeated, continuous, or life threatening, but the prophylactic value of phenytoin is controversial.

   d. Acute hypoglycemia:[10, 11] This condition is commonly encountered up to 30 hours after intoxication, especially in the malnourished, but it may also occur in well-nourished individuals, and mortality may be as high as 11 per cent.

   e. Blood alcohol level:[12, 13] Two studies show increased surgical morbidity when preoperative alcohol levels exceed 250 mg. Excess surgical mortality was not demonstrated.

   f. Cardiac arrhythmias: Hypomagnesemia has been associated with patients who are chronic alcohol abusers. This has been reported by Fisher and Abrams[14] to be associated with ventricular tachyarrhythmias.

   g. Anesthesia: Zaffiri and Francescato[15] have confirmed that more anesthetic was required to overcome the excitatory state in acutely intoxicated humans, but once surgical anesthesia had been established, overall maintenance requirements were reduced because of synergism.

**TABLE 13–19. Signs and Symptoms of Alcohol Withdrawal Syndrome***

| Early (5 to 48 hours) | Late (48 to 96 + hours) |
|---|---|
| Anxiety | Worsening of early symptoms |
| Autonomic hyperactive | |
| increased pulse, blood pressure, respirations | *plus* |
| sweating | |
| tremor | Fever |
| Insomnia | Psychomotor agitation |
| Nightmares | Persistent hallucinations, all sensory modalities |
| Epigastric distress | Delusions |
| anorexia | Disorientation |
| nausea | Delirium |
| vomiting | |
| "butterflies" | |
| Hyperreflexia | |
| Illusions | |
| Transient hallucinations usually visual | |
| insight preserved | |

Minor Withdrawal
Insomnia
Irritability
Tremor

Major Withdrawal
Anxiety
Agitation
Diaphoresis
Disorientation

◄SEIZURES►

DAYS 1 2 3 4 5 6 7

*Tabular material from Leroy JB: Recognition and treatment of the alcohol withdrawal syndrome. Primary Care 6:529, 1974. Diagram from Sellers EM, Kalant H: Alcoholic intoxication and withdrawal. N Engl J Med 294:757, 1976.

  h. Laboratory studies
    (1) CBC with platelets
    (2) Electrolytes, BUN, glucose
    (3) SGOT, SGPT, alkaline phosphatase, bilirubin, albumin
    (4) Amylase
    (5) Prothrombin time and partial thromboplastin time
    (6) Serum calcium, phosphorus, magnesium
    (7) ECG
    (8) Chest x-ray

## B. PERIOPERATIVE MANAGEMENT

  1. Thiamine 100 mg PO, IV, or IM once per day. Should be given before $D_5W$, since Wernicke–Korsakoff syndrome can be precipitated (ophthalmopleglia, ataxia, mental disturbance).
  2. Multivitamins PO or IV once per day
  3. Hydration and replacement of electrolytes
  4. Magnesium replacement can be given after Flink's method, shown in Table 13–20.[16]
  5. Phosphorus replacement can be administered by the following formulas[17] when serum phosphorus levels fall below 1 mg/dl (Table 13–21)

### TABLE 13–20. Suggested Guidelines for Treatment of Magnesium Deficiency

| Day | Dose |
|-----|------|
|     | INTRAMUSCULAR ROUTE (50 % MAGNESIUM SULFATE, SOLUTION) |
| 1   | 2 gm (16.3 mEq) every 2 hours for three doses and then every 4 hours for four doses |
| 2   | 1 gm (8.1 mEq) every 4 hours for six doses |
| 3–5 | 1 gm every 6 hours |
|     | INTRAVENOUS ROUTE (AMPULS OF MAGNESIUM SULFATE) |
| 1   | 6 gm (48 mEq) in 1000-ml solution containing glucose plus any other electrolytes and other medications as indicated. Infuse in 3 hours, followed by 5 gm in each of two 1-liter solutions administered throughout the day. |
| 2   | A total of 6 gm 48 mEq) divided equally in the total fluids of the day |
| 3–5 | Same as Day 2 |

This supplies 32 gm, or 260 mEq, of magnesium.

From Flink EB: Therapy of magnesium deficiency. Ann N Y Acad Sci *162*:901, 1969. Reproduced by permission.

TABLE 13–21. Phosphorus Preparation and Dosages

| Preparation | Phosphate mmol/ml | Phosphorus mg/ml | Na+ | K+ |
|---|---|---|---|---|
| ORAL | | | (mEq/ml) | (mEq/ml) |
| Neutro-phos | 0.107 | 3.33 | 0.095 | 0.095 |
| Phospho-soda | 4.150 | 128.65 | 4.822 | 0 |
| PARENTERAL | | | | |
| Na phosphate | 0.090 | 2.8 | 0.161 | 0 |
| Na, K phosphate | 0.100 | 3.10 | 0.162 | 0.019 |

    a. Recent or uncomplicated hypophosphatemia: 2.5 mg/kg (0.08 mmol/kg) over six hours; then recheck phosphorus level for further dosing

    b. Prolonged or multiple causes for hypophosphatemia: 5 mg/kg (0.16 mmol/kg) over six hours; then recheck phosphorus level for further dosing. Do not exceed 7.5 mg/kg (0.24 mmol/kg)

6. Management of withdrawal symptoms[2, 18,19] (Table 13–22)

7. Seizures

    If seizures should occur and are recurrent, the following phenytoin dosage schedule is used:

    a. IV: 15 to 18 mg/kg loading dose; then 4 to 8 mg/kg/day maintenance

    b. PO: 400 mg—300 mg—300 mg at two-hour intervals

8. Alcohol

    Gower and Kerstein[20] recommend IV alcohol to allow a necessary procedure to be performed and then manage the alcohol withdrawal process. The recommended dosage is 5 per cent ethanol in 1 liter of dextrose and water titrated to the patient's signs and symptoms.

TABLE 13–22. Drug Therapy for Alcohol Withdrawal Symptoms

| Clinical State* | Drug | Dose | Interval | Route |
|---|---|---|---|---|
| Extreme agitation | Diazepam | 5 mg | q 5 min until calm; then q6h | IV |
| Mild to moderate agitation, anxiety, tremor | Chlordiazepoxide | 25–100 mg | q 6 hrs | PO |
| | Diazepam | 5 mg–20 mg | q 6 hrs | PO |

*The clinical status of the patient must be checked routinely to assess ongoing dosage amount and frequency.

## REFERENCES

1. Leroy JB: Recognition and treatment of the alcohol withdrawal syndrome. Primary Care 6:529, 1974.
2. Sellers EM, Kalant H: Alcoholic intoxication and withdrawal. N Engl J Med 294:757, 1976.
3. Victor M: Treatment of alcoholic intoxication and the withdrawal syndrome: A critical analysis of the use of drugs and other forms of therapy. Psychosom Med 28:636, 1966.
4. Hotmann FG: A Handbook on Drug and Alcohol Abuse. New York, Oxford Press, 1975.
5. Kissin B: Medical management of the alcoholic patient, in Kissin B, Begleiter H (eds): Treatment and Rehabilitation of the Chronic Alcoholic. The Biology of Alcoholism. New York, Plenum Press, 1977, vol 5, p 55.
6. Victor M, Wolfe SM: Causation and treatment of the alcohol withdrawal syndrome, in Bourne PG, Fox R (eds): Alcoholism: Progress in Research and Treatment. New York, Academic Press, 1973, p 137.
7. Victor M, Adams RD: The effect of alcohol on the nervous system. Res Publ Assoc Res Nerv Ment Dis 32:526, 1953.
8. Sampliner RE, Iber FL: Diphenylhydantoin control of alcohol withdrawal seizures: Results of a controlled study. JAMA 230:1430, 1974.
9. Wolfe SM, Victor M: The relationship of hypomagnesemia and alkalosis to alcohol withdrawal symptoms. Ann NY Acad Sci 62:973, 1969.
10. Madison LL: Ethanol-induced hypoglycemia. Adv Metab Disord 3:85, 1968.
11. Arky RA, Freinkel NI. In Sardesi VM (ed): Biochemical and Clinical Aspects of Alcohol Metabolism. Springfield, Charles C Thomas, 1969, p 67.
12. Lee JF, Giescke AJ, Jenkins MT: Anesthetic management of trauma: Influence of alcohol ingestion. South Med J 60:1240, 1967.
13. Lee JF, Samuelson RJ, Watson TD, Giescke AJ: Anesthesia for trauma: Is blood alcohol level a factor? Tex Med 7:84, 1974.
14. Fisher J, Abrams J: Life-threatening ventricular tachyarrhythmias in delirium tremens. JAMA 137:1238, 1977.
15. Zaffiri O, Francescato F: Problemi anestesiologici nell' alcoolisma acuto. Minerva Anestesio 33:263, 1967.
16. Flink EB: Therapy of magnesium deficiency. Ann NY Acad Sci 162:901, 1969.
17. Lentz RD, Brown DM, Kjellstrand CM: Treatment of severe hypophosphatemia. Ann Intern Med 89:941, 1978.
18. Thompson WL: Management of alcohol withdrawal syndromes. Arch Intern Med 138:278, 1978.
19. Thompson WL, Johnson AD, Maddrey WC: Diazepam and paraldehyde for treatment of severe delirium tremens. Ann Intern Med 82:175, 1975.
20. Gower WE, Kerstein H: Prevention of alcohol withdrawal symptoms in surgical patients. Surg Gynecol Obstet 151:382, 1980.

# INDEX

Page numbers in *italics* indicate illustrations; page numbers followed by t indicate tables.